Diabetes
COOKBOOK

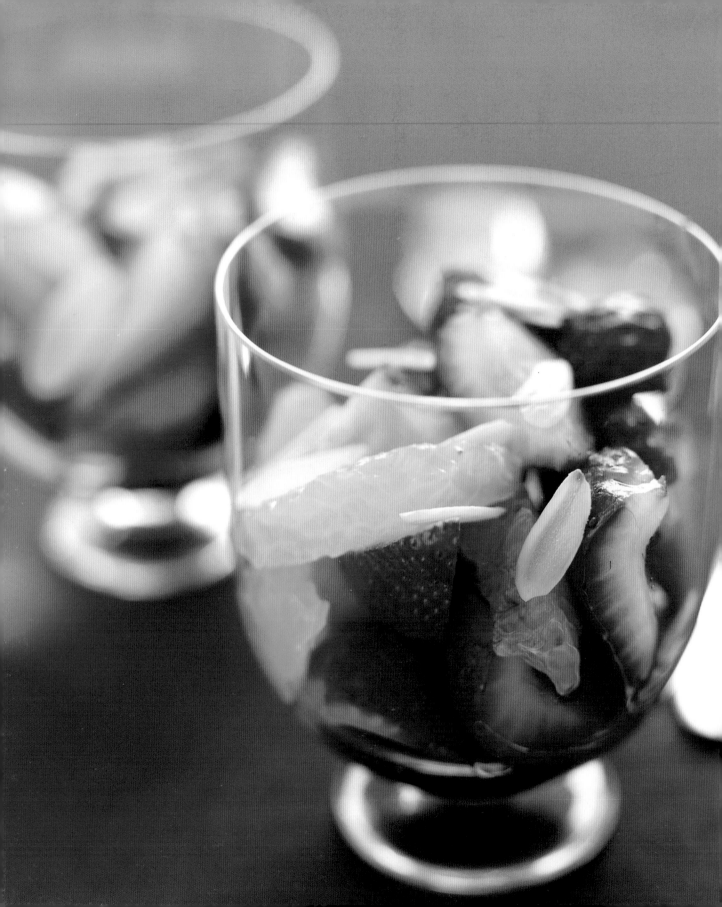

AMERICAN MEDICAL ASSOCIATION

Diabetes
COOKBOOK

641.56

RECIPES
Maureen Callahan, R.D.
Karen A. Levin

PHOTOGRAPHS
Jim Franco
Sheri Giblin

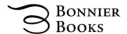

BONNIER
BOOKS

CONTENTS

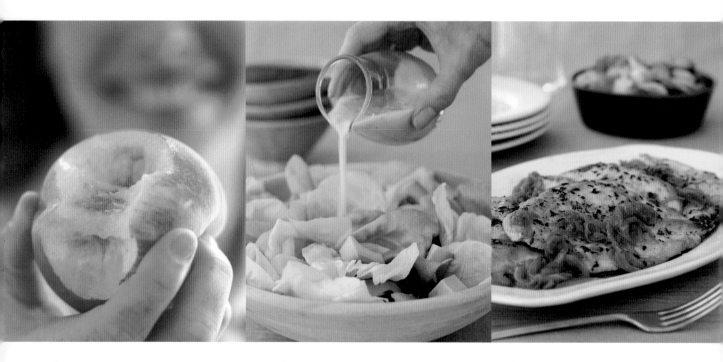

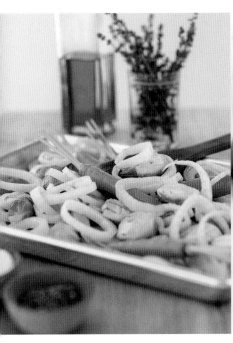
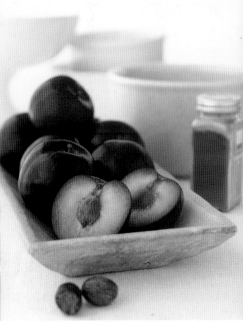
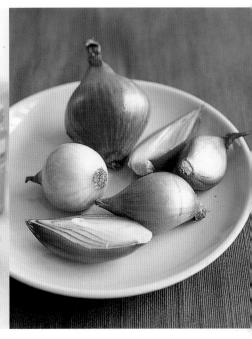

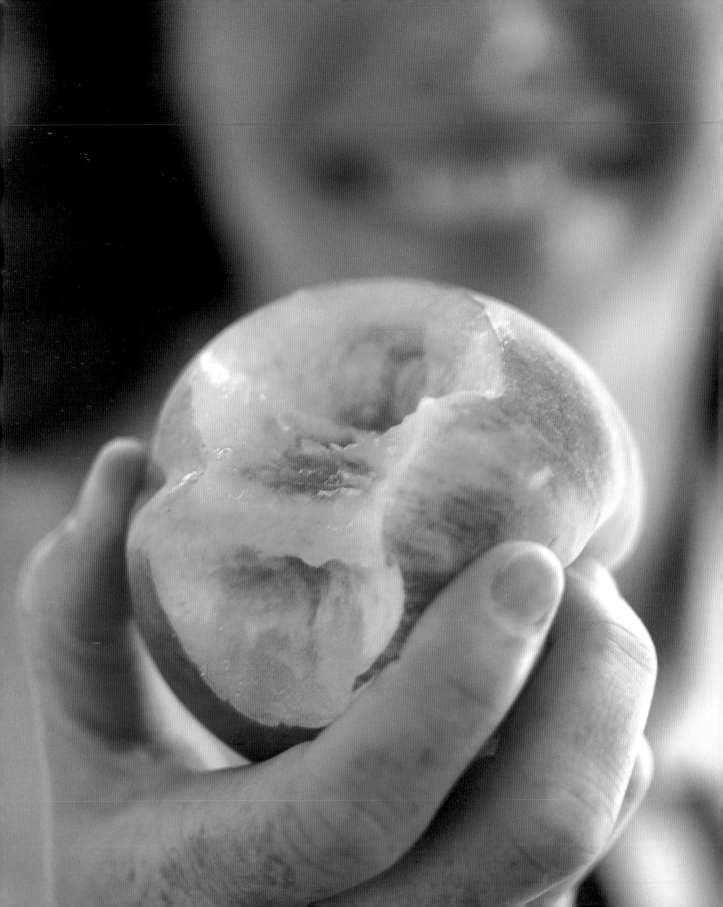

LIVING WELL WITH DIABETES

EATING IS ONE OF LIFE'S GREATEST PLEASURES, AND EATING WELL IS ONE OF THE MOST IMPORTANT THINGS YOU CAN DO FOR YOUR HEALTH. EVERY DAY, RESEARCHERS DISCOVER A NEW LINK BETWEEN DIET AND HEALTH. If you are one of the thousands of Britons who have diabetes, choosing the right foods may sometimes seem like a chore. Although it's true that if you have diabetes you need to carefully balance the food you eat with your physical activity to keep your blood glucose at a healthy level, eating does not have to be a burden. With only a small amount of planning and preparation and the delicious recipes you'll find in this cookbook, you can eat just as well as anyone else and enjoy food just as much.

The American Medical Association has developed this diverse collection of recipes with you in mind, whether you have diabetes or have been warned that you're at risk of developing it – or whether you simply want to eat more healthily. The sixty dishes in this book are not only tasty, but also attractive and quick and easy to prepare. They're designed by nutrition professionals to help you stay in good health while making everyday eating a pleasurable part of life for you and your family.

UNDERSTANDING DIABETES

If you have diabetes, your doctor and diabetes adviser or dietitian have helped you develop a nutrition plan. If you have been told your blood-sugar level puts you at risk of developing diabetes, your doctor has no doubt recommended steps you can take to reduce this risk. It pays, however, to remember the facts about the two main forms of diabetes.

CONTROL YOUR BLOOD SUGAR

Keeping your blood-sugar level in the range your doctor has set for you can help you prevent or slow complications from diabetes. Here are some helpful tips:

• Eat about the same amount of food every day.

• Eat meals and snacks at about the same time each day.

• Don't skip meals or snacks.

• Take your diabetes medicine at the same time every day.

• Try to exercise at about the same time each day.

Disease-fighting foods (facing page, clockwise from top left): haricot beans, high in fibre and protein; rocket, a flavourful green high in antioxidants; salmon, a source of heart-healthy Omega-3 fatty acids; and a salad with vitamin-rich spinach and beetroot.

Type 1 diabetes

Type 1 diabetes usually develops during childhood when the pancreas stops producing insulin or doesn't produce it in sufficient quantity, causing sugar to build up in the blood. Type 1 diabetes is much less common than Type 2; only about 5 to 10 per cent of people with diabetes have this form. To stay healthy, people with Type 1 diabetes must follow a carefully controlled diet and have daily injections of insulin throughout life to keep their blood-sugar level in a normal range.

Type 2 diabetes

Of the thousands of Britons with diabetes, 90 to 95 per cent have Type 2, which is becoming an epidemic throughout the world and striking increasing numbers of children.

Type 2 diabetes develops from an interaction of genes and lifestyle factors, especially lack of exercise and excess weight, which cause the body to stop responding to the effects of insulin, a hormone that enables the body to use sugar for energy.

Unlike Type 1 diabetes, Type 2 diabetes can sometimes be prevented and controlled with measures such as regular exercise and weight loss.

Blood-sugar's role

Sugar is the fuel that energizes all the cells of the body, but excess sugar in the blood makes some components of the blood "sticky" and the blood vessels more likely to develop fatty deposits that can build up and reduce or block blood flow. The damage to blood vessels and nerves from excess sugar in the blood over time can lead to serious long-term complications, including vision loss, kidney disease, stroke from high blood pressure, and heart disease.

People who have precise control of their blood sugar are much less likely to experience these complications – all the more reason to consistently follow the recommendations of your doctor and diabetes adviser.

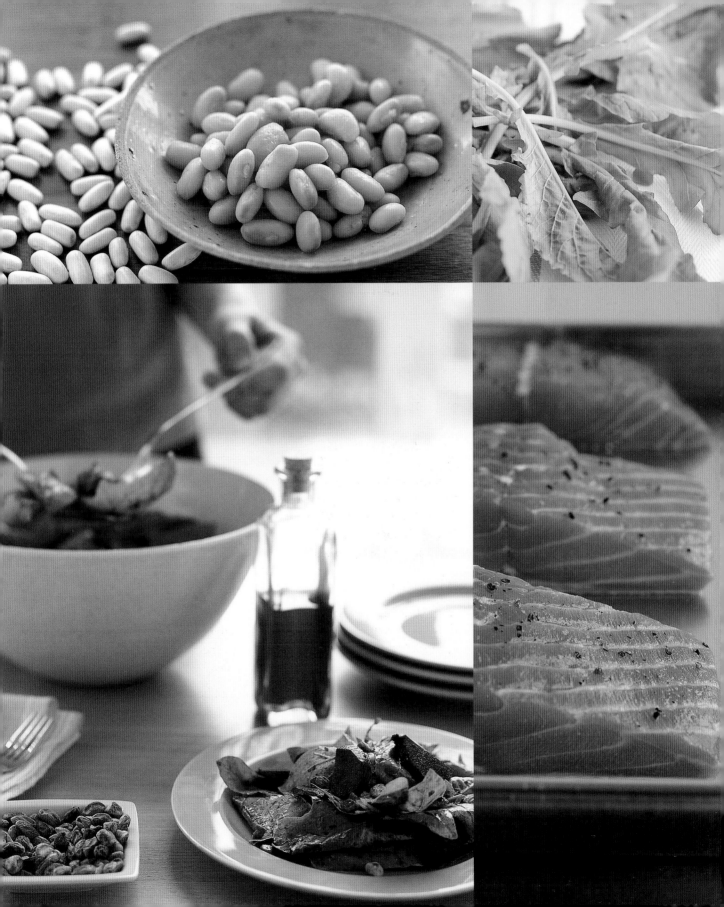

MANAGING YOUR DIABETES

Your blood-sugar level depends on factors such as your diet, weight, activity, and medications – even your emotions. If you have Type 1 diabetes, you will probably be most concerned about balancing your food intake with your insulin dosages and exercise. If you have Type 2, you may be more interested in weight control.

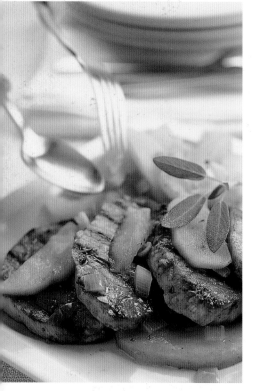

Low-fat dishes such as Pork Loin with Apples (page 74) fit well in diabetic diets if balanced with whole grains, beans, and greens.

Biking and walking (facing page) are simple activities that can help people with diabetes control their blood sugar and weight.

Watch your diet

Diet is a major factor in controlling blood-sugar levels, but there is no standard diabetic diet that works for everyone.

What diabetic meal plans have in common is that they are based on scientific understanding of the nutrient needs of the human body. They are heart-healthy, calorie-conscious, high in fibre and other important nutrients, and low in harmful fats and sweets. Specifically, they are rich in whole grains, vegetables, pulses, and fruit, and they replace unhealthy fats (such as those in fatty meats) with healthy plant-based fats (such as olive oil) and Omega-3 fatty acids (from fish).

Work with your doctor or dietitian to develop a personal nutrition plan designed to provide essential nutrients and help you maintain a healthy weight. The recipes in this book can be part of your plan, helping you control your blood-sugar levels while you enjoy satifying meals.

Stay at a healthy weight

Obesity, which is widespread in Britain and increasing, is one of the major factors contributing to the epidemic of Type 2 diabetes. Losing weight can help you prevent Type 2 diabetes or, if you already have diabetes, can reduce the severity of the disease by making your body more sensitive to insulin. Even a moderate weight loss – 4.5 kilograms (10 pounds) or so – can reduce your blood sugar and benefit your health.

No miracle diet exists. If you want to lose weight and keep the weight off, you have to consume fewer calories than your body burns. Avoid diets that claim otherwise.

Because managing your diabetes with drugs or insulin can sometimes cause weight gain, avoid overeating and strive to make exercise a part of every day. Above all, work closely with your doctor and diabetes adviser to develop a safe and effective weight-loss plan that is tailored to your daily life.

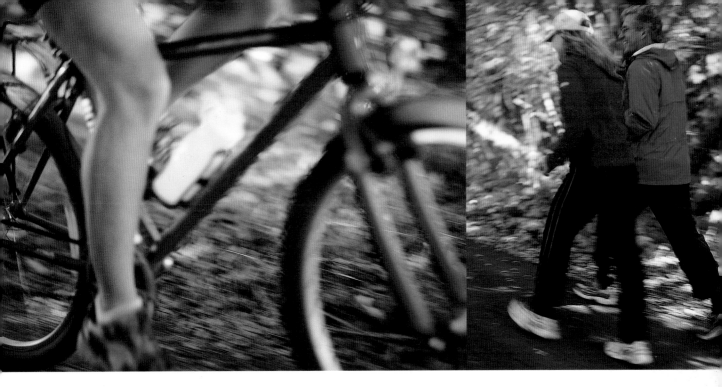

Get moving

Exercise helps you control your blood sugar by making your body more sensitive to insulin, promoting weight loss, and reducing fat around your abdomen. Exercise also lowers blood pressure, reduces your risk of heart disease, improves blood cholesterol levels, and relieves stress.

Try to engage in regular physical activity for 30 to 60 minutes every day. Walking is the form of exercise that doctors recommend most.

Talk with your doctor about the types of physical activity that are best for you. He or she might recommend precautions such as testing your blood glucose before and after exercise and watching for signs of low blood sugar during and after exercise.

Manage your medication

If diet, weight loss, and exercise are not enough to keep your blood-sugar level in an acceptable range, your doctor will prescribe a sugar-lowering medication or insulin.

The type of medication you take depends on many factors, including your age, the severity of your diabetes, other health issues, and other medications you are taking. (Some drugs reduce the effectiveness of some diabetes medications.)

Even if you are taking a diabetes medication, a healthy diet and regular exercise are key to managing your condition. Your medication works together with your diet and your exercise programme – it doesn't replace them.

CHECK YOUR BLOOD SUGAR

The best way to make sure your blood sugar is in a safe range is to check it frequently.

If you take insulin, your doctor has told you how many times a day you should check your blood sugar. Frequent testing helps you evaluate how well your diet, exercise, and medication are working.

A glycohaemoglobin test, performed in the doctor's office or at home, helps your doctor tell how well your diabetes has been controlled over the past few months.

Keep in mind, however, that routine haemoglobin tests are not a substitute for daily blood-glucose testing at home.

SETTING NUTRITION GOALS

Although there is no one-size-fits-all diabetic diet, certain healthy eating guidelines apply to everyone who has diabetes. The recipes in this book will help you follow these guidelines.

Because people who have diabetes are at risk of developing heart disease, you need to do more than control your blood-sugar levels to stay healthy. Consume a balanced diet that is low in calories, saturated and trans fats, salt, sugar, and alcohol. Choose whole grains over refined ones and add high-fibre vegetables, fruit, and pulses.

The food you eat is composed of carbohydrates, fats, and protein. Carbohydrates and fats are your body's main sources of fuel. Carbs should make up 45 to 65 per cent of your daily calories, fats (primarily from vegetable fats) about 20 to 35 per cent, and protein about 12 to 20 per cent.

HOW TO DISTRIBUTE YOUR DAILY CALORIES

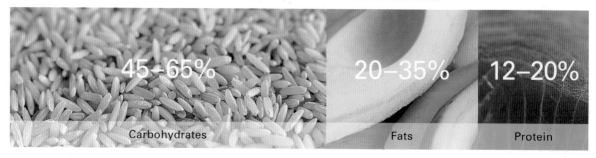

45–65%	20–35%	12–20%
Carbohydrates	Fats	Protein

CARBOHYDRATES

Carbohydrates are the sugars, starches, and fibre that make up foods such as grains, fruit, and vegetables. The total amount of carbohydrate in a meal or snack matters more than whether it's sugar or starch. If you take insulin, adjust the dose before a meal based on how much carbohydrate you plan to eat, because carbohydrates can raise blood sugar quickly.

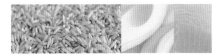

45–65% OF DAILY CALORIES FROM CARBS

Sugars

Sugars found in many foods include fructose and sucrose (in fruit) and lactose (in milk). Granulated sugar and high-fructose golden syrup are often added to foods and drinks. Sweets do not raise blood sugar faster than do some starches, but they contain few nutrients and little fibre.

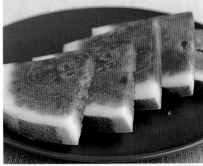

Starches

Starches are carbohydrates in bread, grains, cereal, pasta, sweetcorn, squash, and potatoes. Wholegrain starches are healthier than refined ones because they provide more vitamins, minerals, and fibre. They also help keep blood sugar steady.

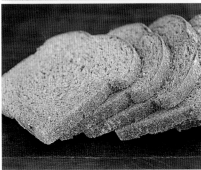

Fibre

Fibre, the indigestible part of plant food, plays a special role in healthy diets. Soluble fibre – found in oats, pulses, barley, and certain fruit and vegetables – not only reduces blood-sugar levels but also improves blood-cholesterol levels.

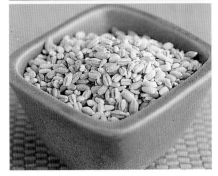

ARTIFICIAL SWEETENERS

Carb-free and mostly calorie-free alternatives to sugar can be found in these artificial sweeteners:

ASPARTAME The most widely used sugar substitute, aspartame is 180 times sweeter than sugar. People who cannot tolerate phenyl-alanine should avoid aspartame.

ACESULPHAME-K Also known as acesulphame potassium, acesulph-ame-K is found in baked goods, drinks, frozen desserts, and sweets.

SUCRALOSE Sucralose is made from sugar but cannot be digested, so it adds no calories and does not affect blood-glucose levels. It is 600 times sweeter than sugar.

CYCLAMATE Cyclamate (E952), 30–50 times sweeter than sugar, is mainly used in dilutable soft drinks.

SACCHARIN Although saccharin faced a proposed ban in 1977 because of a possible link to cancer in animals, it remains on the market. Moderate use is considered safe.

HEALTHY FATS

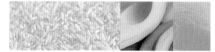

Fats in food help your body store energy and transport some vitamins through the bloodstream. They make food taste smooth and creamy and help make you feel full. Oils from nuts, seeds, and vegetables, as well as fats from fish, provide health benefits and can reduce your risk of heart disease. These fats, known as unsaturated fats, are usually liquid.

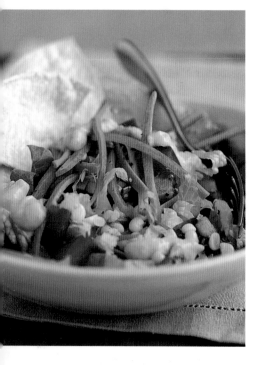

Heart-healthy fats from avocado add rich creaminess to the dressing for Chopped Salad with Lime-Avocado Dressing (page 49).

Monounsaturated fats

Olive, sunflower, and peanut oils are the main sources of mono-unsaturated fats, the healthiest fats you can eat. They lower LDL (the so-called bad cholesterol) and raise HDL (good cholesterol) in the blood, helping lower heart-disease risk.

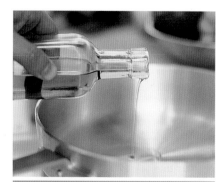

Polyunsaturated fats

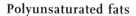

These fats, essential for good health, include corn, sunflower, safflower, linseed, and soya bean oils, as well as the oils in fatty fish such as salmon. Rich in Omega-3 and Omega-6 fatty acids, they lower total cholesterol but also cut HDL (good) cholesterol.

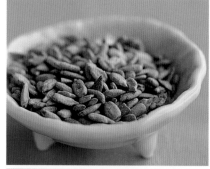

Plant sterols

Nuts, seeds, and many other plant foods contain substances called plant sterols that slow the absorption of dietary cholesterol and can lower LDL (bad) and total cholesterol levels in the blood. Soft margarines and salad dressings with added plant sterols are available in most stores.

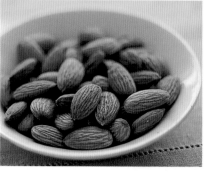

HARMFUL FATS

Not all types of fat are healthy. Saturated and trans fats can increase your risk of heart disease and some forms of cancer. These fats are usually solid or semisolid at room temperature, although they may turn liquid when heated. It's not possible to avoid all harmful fats because they occur in many foods, but it's best to cut back wherever you can.

Saturated fats

Plentiful in meat, dark meat poultry and poultry skin, butter, full-fat dairy products, coconut oil, and palm oil, saturated fats increase total blood cholesterol and LDL (bad) cholesterol. Limit these fats, along with trans fats, to no more than 8 to 10 per cent of your total daily calories.

Trans fats

Block margarine and white vegetable fats contain hydrogenated oils that raise total blood cholesterol and LDL (bad) cholesterol levels. These so-called trans fats are common in packaged and processed foods, baked goods, and fried foods such as chips.

Cholesterol

Egg yolks, liver, shellfish, and full-fat dairy products are rich in cholesterol, which can raise blood cholesterol, although it does not do so in all people. Saturated and trans fats have a greater impact on blood cholesterol than does dietary cholesterol.

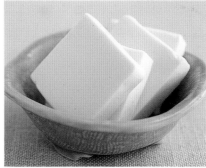
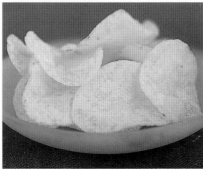
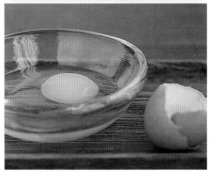

FIGURING YOUR FAT

When you are figuring your daily intake of fat (which should be about 30 per cent of your total calories each day), consider the total amount of fat eaten during the day, not just in one meal. If you have a big, rich breakfast, for example, limit the amount of fat in your lunch or dinner that day. Here are some other tips:

• Limit fatty meats, full-fat dairy products, and rich baked goods.

• Choose foods made with healthy plant-based fats, such as avocados, olive and sunflower oils, and nuts.

• Limit your cholesterol intake to less than 300 milligrams a day, or 200 mg if you have heart disease.

• Make some meals meatless.

PROTEIN

12–20% OF DAILY CALORIES FROM PROTEIN

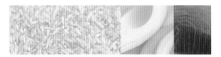

Protein, an essential nutrient found in both plant and animal foods, repairs tissues, builds muscle, and carries hormones and vitamins throughout the body via the bloodstream. Infants and growing children have the highest daily protein requirements, but most Americans consume far more protein than they actually need.

HOW MUCH PROTEIN IS ENOUGH?

Adults need a surprisingly small quantity of protein every day – only 0.8 g of protein per kilogram (2.2 lb) of body weight.

There are almost 30 g of protein in a 75-g (3-oz) chicken breast and in a 500-ml (18-fl oz) bowl of bean soup. Use your weight to determine how much protein you may need in a day using the chart below:

60 kg	—	48 grams
65 kg	—	52 grams
70 kg	—	56 grams
75 kg	—	60 grams
80 kg	—	64 grams

Some people with diabetes have advanced kidney disease and need to limit their daily protein intake to 0.6 g per kilogram of body weight. To monitor your kidneys' health, your doctor will recommend regular kidney-function tests.

Red meat and poultry

Beef, pork, lamb, chicken, and turkey are protein-rich foods that often contain large amounts of harmful saturated fats (page 15), although lean cuts are available. The portions of foods such as beef and chicken in this cookbook are relatively small.

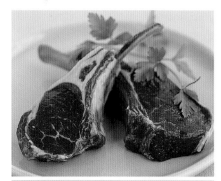

Pulses and fish

Plant proteins such as beans, lentils, peas, and nuts contain healthier fats than do animal proteins, have no cholesterol, and provide healthy fibre. Fish, also a fine protein source, has about as much protein as lean beef, gram for gram, but also supplies heart-healthy Omega-3 fatty acids.

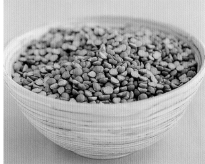

High-protein diets

Low-carbohydrate, high-protein, high-fat diets can result in rapid weight loss but may cause kidney problems for some people with diabetes. Talk to your doctor and nutritionist if you are thinking about trying a high-protein diet.

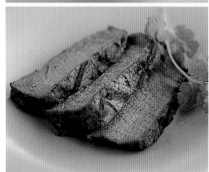

SALT

For some people, consuming too much salt raises blood pressure. High blood pressure is a major risk factor for heart disease and other complications to which people with diabetes are especially vulnerable.

Going low sodium

If you have high blood pressure, your doctor may have asked you to lower your intake of salt. But limiting salt means more than just putting away the salt shaker. It also means staying away from most fast foods and highly salted packaged and tinned foods, such as soups and vegetables and the flavour packets that come with many packaged dishes.

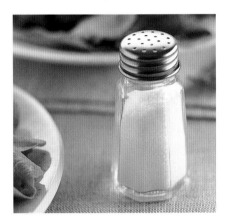

ALCOHOL

Although moderate drinking can reduce heart-attack risk, doctors don't recommend drinking for your health. People with diabetes need to be careful because alcohol interferes with the liver's production of sugar.

Alcohol's impact on blood sugar

If you drink alcohol while taking a diabetes drug that lowers blood sugar or on an empty stomach, your blood sugar could drop dangerously low, and it can remain low for 24 hours, even after just one drink. At other times, the carbs in an alcoholic drink, especially when mixed with something sweet, can raise blood sugar too high.

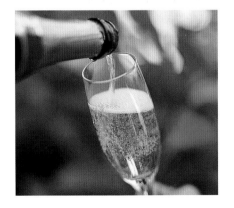

COUNTING CARBOHYDRATES

Because carbohydrates are the main influence on blood sugar, your doctor may suggest keeping track of the grams of carbohydrates you eat each day. This method is newer than using food exchanges, although exchanges are still widely used. How many daily carbohydrate grams are right for you? Follow the three easy steps in the next few pages to estimate your allowance.

HOW TO FIND THE NUTRIENT VALUES IN EACH RECIPE

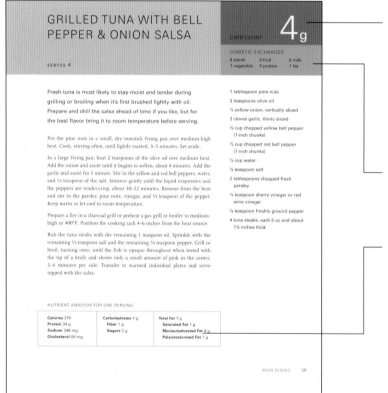

Carb Count At the top of each recipe page you'll see a prominent number labelled "Carb Count", the number of grams (g) of carbohydrate in one serving of the dish. To find recipes listed by their carb counts, turn to the start of each recipe chapter (pages 27, 53, 95, and 117). Use the counts to plan healthy menus (page 22).

Diabetic Exchanges This box offers details on each recipe for people using the conventional food-exchange system, explained in the box on page 19.

Nutrient Analysis At the bottom of the page find the recipe's fats, calories, and other key nutrients, calculated by a registered dietitian. Each recipe is low in calories, harmful fats, cholesterol, and sodium, and many are high in fibre. Along with nutrition facts from packaged foods, these numbers can help you plan well-balanced meals. Measures are in grams (g) and milligrams (mg). They have been rounded to the nearest whole number.

1 NOTE YOUR ACTIVITY LEVEL

Your activity level and weight together determine the amount of food you can eat. The more frequent and intense your activities, the more food energy – calories – you burn. Of course, everyday activities such as shopping take less energy than exercise such as jogging. Read the descriptions below to find the one that best describes your activity level.

Take your activity level and go to step 2 →

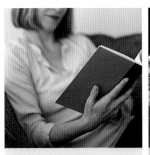

INACTIVE

Mainly sedentary most days of the week. Daily activities limited to driving, reading, watching television, and cooking, with only rare, light exertion such as shopping.

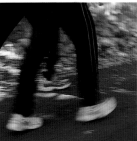

SOMEWHAT ACTIVE

Low-intensity activity throughout the week. Activities include light housework, leisurely walks, playing with children, climbing stairs at home, low-intensity sports, such as golf or bowling.

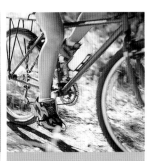

ACTIVE

Vigorous exercise several days a week. Activities include long brisk walks or bike rides, gardening, mid-intensity sports, such as tennis, skiing, cricket, swimming, dancing, or yoga.

DIABETIC EXCHANGES

The food-exchange system – an alternative way for people with diabetes to plan meals – breaks each serving into nutrients of concern, such as starch, sugar or other carbs, fat, and protein.

Food-exchange lists may also show whether the serving contains significant ingredients in the fruit, vegetable, milk, or protein food groups (as shown in this book).

Each exchange is a portion of food that has about the same number of calories as another in its group. In the starch group, for example, 85 g (3 oz) of sweetcorn is the same as half a muffin. Both would be rated "1 starch" in the Diabetic Exchanges box. That means you can exchange one for the other and keep your calories about the same.

People recently diagnosed with diabetes typically consult with a dietitian and receive daily exchange targets based on their blood-sugar levels and daily calorie needs.

Activity's benefits

Regular exercise can help you control your blood-sugar level. What's more, less-active people who increase their activity even a little reap many benefits, including improved cholesterol levels, lower blood pressure, sounder sleep more upbeat mood, increased alertness, and improved memory – and they tend to lose weight. Talk to your doctor or diabetes adviser about the right activity for you.

2 FIND YOUR CALORIE NEEDS

The more you weigh, the more calories you need to consume every day. To determine how many calories you can eat each day without gaining or losing pounds, find your weight on the far left side of the chart below; then locate your daily calorie allowance to the right in the column that corresponds to your activity level.

Take your calorie needs and go to step 3 →

LOSE WEIGHT SAFELY

People with diabetes who lose excess weight can improve their blood sugar and have better control of their diabetes. To lose a pound a week – a safe goal – it's necessary to cut about 500 calories a day.

A good approach is to cut back on high-fat, high-sugar, and high-sodium foods and to plan more meals and snacks around whole grains, vegetables, and fruit.

An apple and a chocolate bar both contain about 30 grams of carbohydrate, but the apple is nearly fat free while the chocolate has 15 grams of fat and 150 more calories.

WEIGHT (kg)	INACTIVE	SOMEWHAT ACTIVE	ACTIVE
55	1500	1700	1800
60	1600	1800	1900
60	1700	1900	2100
70	1800	2000	2200
73	2000	2100	2400
77	2100	2300	2500
82	2200	2400	2700
85	2300	2500	2800
90	2500	2700	3000
95	2600	2800	3100
100	2700	3000	3300
105	2800	3100	3400
110	2900	3200	3600
115	3100	3300	3700
120	3200	3500	3900
125	3300	3600	4000
130	3400	3700	4100

CALORIES

3 LOCATE YOUR CARB COUNT

For most people, carbohydrates should make up about 55 per cent of their total daily calories. However, your doctor may recommend a lower or higher percentage (see What's Your Carb Percentage? below right). In the chart below, find the box with your daily calorie allowance to find the number of grams (g) of carbohydrate you can eat each day.

To use your carb count turn the page →

CALORIES	CARBS	CALORIES	CARBS	CALORIES	CARBS
1500	210g	2400	330g	3300	455g
1600	220g	2500	345g	3400	470g
1700	235g	2600	360g	3500	480g
1800	250g	2700	370g	3600	495g
1900	260g	2800	385g	3700	510g
2000	275g	2900	400g	3800	525g
2100	290g	3000	415g	3900	540g
2200	300g	3100	425g	4000	550g
2300	315g	3200	440g	4100	565g

WHAT'S YOUR CARB PERCENTAGE?

Because carbohydrates have a greater effect on blood sugar than do other nutrients, your doctor may ask you to adjust the percentage of carbs in your diet. The chart at left shows the number of carb grams that equal 55 per cent of total daily calories. If your doctor or diabetes adviser has suggested eating less or more, use the following easy formula. If your daily calorie need is 1800 and your carb per cent is 45:

1 Multiply 1800 by 0.45. That equals 810 carb calories per day.

2 Divide your daily carb calories by 4 (the number of calories in 1 g of carbohydrate). Your daily carb count is 202 g.

PLANNING HEALTHY MENUS

Planning menus can be time-consuming when you have diabetes. To help keep your blood sugar steady, it's important to divide up your daily carb count and spread your carb grams throughout the day. You have to measure portions, time your meals, track carbs, and balance it all with exercise and medication. Here's a plan using recipes in this book.

A sample day's menu

Say your carb count is 260 g and your dietitian has suggested you spread them between three meals and a snack – 30 per cent for each meal and 10 per cent for the snack.

Breakfast (per serving)	**78 g**
Pineapple Smoothie (page 128)	38 g
Blueberry Bran Muffin (page 132)	26 g
250 ml (18 fl oz) skimmed milk	14 g
Lunch (per serving)	**78 g**
Bean Tostada (page 88)	41 g
Chopped Salad with Lime-Avocado Dressing (page 49)	28 g
9 fresh strawberries	9 g
Snack (per serving)	**26 g**
12 Spicy Pitta Crisps (page 133)	26 g
Dinner (per serving)	**78 g**
Spinach & Garlic Lasagne (page 84)	39 g
Roasted Winter Vegetables (page 115)	14 g
Balsamic-Glazed Berries & Tangerines (page 127)	25 g
Day's total	**260 g**

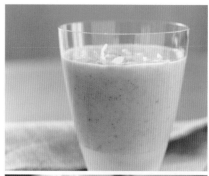

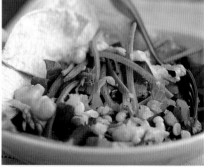

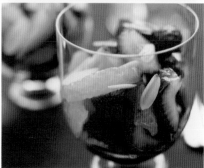

COOKING FOR GOOD HEALTH

Having healthy ingredients on hand – like low-sodium tinned stock and tomatoes in the larder, and lean meats and wholegrain bread in the freezer – allows you to put together nutritious meals quickly and easily.

Variety is key

Keep your meals simple but vary your diet by trying new grains, fruit, and vegetables. Experiment with vegetarian dishes. Vegetarians are less likely than meat-eaters to develop heart disease, high blood pressure, and obesity, making a meatless diet especially beneficial for people with diabetes. But you need to plan vegetarian meals carefully to ensure that you get sufficient protein and other essential nutrients.

Smart shopping

Take advantage of the many reduced-fat, fat-free, low-sodium, and sugar-free products now on sale. Stock plenty of fresh, frozen, and tinned vegetables and fruit (without added sugar). Seek out unsweetened high-fibre cereals and low-fat cheese. Shop for salt-free "natural" peanut butter, not fatty and salty convenience foods. Check labels to find low-fat foods containing 3 g of fat or fewer for every 100 calories.

Healthier choices in the kitchen

You know it's wise to choose low-fat dairy products over full-fat ones and whole grains over refined ones. Try these other healthy options.

Replace minced meat with beans or soya protein.

Substitute 2 egg whites for each whole egg.

Use soya milk or rice milk instead of cow's milk.

Replace butter, bacon fat, and lard with sunflower, olive, or peanut oil.

Use lemon juice or vinegar and herbs and spices in place of salt.

Whip evaporated skimmed milk instead of double cream.

Substitute soft tofu for ricotta cheese.

Marinate poultry and meat in low-fat yoghurt instead of oil.

WHAT'S A SERVING?

Serving sizes can be confusing. For example, a juice carton may say a serving is 250 ml (8 fl oz), while your recommended serving size is 125 ml (4 fl oz). Here are some tips for watching how much you eat:

• Use measuring spoons for accuracy and weigh all foods on a scale. Do not use guesswork.

• Weigh bread slices and bagel halves to make sure they fit into your carb count. If they're too large, cut them into smaller pieces.

• Divide and weigh meat and poultry portions before cooking. A 75-g (3-oz) piece should fit in your palm.

FOODS THAT FIGHT DIABETES

INGREDIENT	CONTAINS	HEALTH BENEFIT
Oats • pulses • vegetables • dried fruit • whole grains • berries and other fresh fruit	**Fibre**	Help control weight; promotes healthy digestion; soluble fibre improves cholesterol and lowers blood sugar.
Fruit and vegetables • nuts • vegetable oils • wheat germ • fish and seafood	**Antioxidants**	Fight cell-damaging free radicals, which are produced when blood sugar is high and may contribute to complications of diabetes.
Nuts and seeds • corn oil and soya bean oil • soft margarines with added sterols	**Plant sterols**	Lower cholesterol levels.
Pulses • fish • poultry • lean meats • low-fat dairy products • low-fat tofu	**Low-fat protein**	Build, maintain, and repair body tissues.
Salmon • sardines • mackerel • herring • linseed and linseed oil	**Omega-3 fatty acids**	Reduce heart disease risk by improving cholesterol and preventing blood clots; reduce joint pain and inflammation.
Dark green leafy vegetables • fruit • pulses • wheat germ • whole grains	**Folic acid**	Reduces heart risk by reducing homocysteine in the blood; helps form blood cells; essential in pregnancy for preventing birth defects.

INGREDIENT	CONTAINS	HEALTH BENEFIT
Onions and garlic • chives • shallots • leeks	Allicin	A sulphur-containing substance that may lower cholesterol, reduce blood-clotting, and control blood pressure.
Dairy products • fortified juices • fortified breakfast cereals • pulses • tinned fish (with bones)	Calcium	Essential for transmitting nerve impulses, regulating heart rhythm, and enhancing muscle function; maintains bone strength.
Bran cereals • whole grains • green beans • broccoli • spices • processed meats	Chromium	Enhance insulin's effects in converting sugar, protein, and fat into energy; works with insulin to transport sugar from the blood into cells.
Spinach and beet greens • nuts • whole grains • pulses • dairy products • fish • meat • poultry	Magnesium	Help lower blood pressure; help prevent irregular heartbeat; more is needed when blood sugar is high and when taking diuretics.
Whole grains • sunflower seeds • oysters • gelatin • vegetable oil • sweetcorn • parsley • green beans • soya	Vanadium	A trace mineral that promotes insulin production and increases the body's sensitivity to insulin.
Shellfish • red meat • pulses • nuts • eggs • tofu and other soya foods • wheat germ	Zinc	Needed for the breakdown of protein, fat, and carbohydrates; helps make protein and insulin; essential for growth and development.

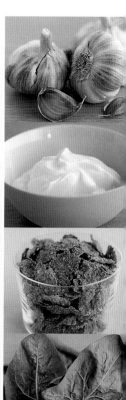

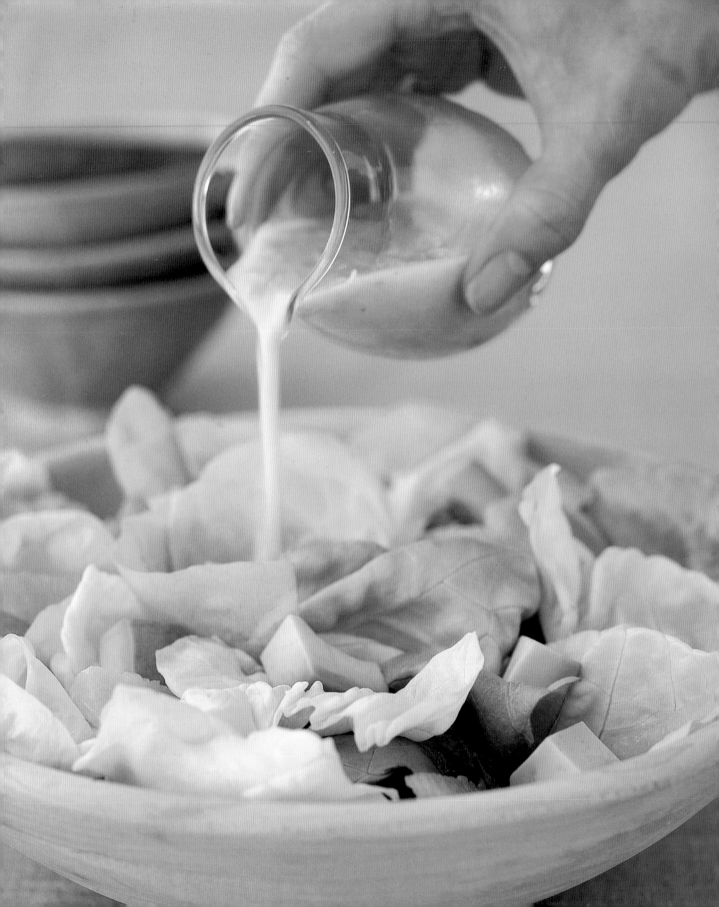

STARTERS, SOUPS & SALADS

Lettuce Salad with Orange & Avocado, 45

RED PEPPER QUESADILLAS

SERVES 4

1½ teaspoons olive oil or sunflower oil

½ diced red sweet pepper

2 spring onions, thinly sliced

2 tablespoons chopped fresh coriander

2 mild green chillies, seeded and chopped

8 corn tortillas, 15 cm (6 in) in diameter

40 g (1½ oz) Monterey Jack cheese or Cheddar cheese, grated

These toasty quesadillas can be mild or spicy—simply vary the amount of chilli you add. For an extra-light version, replace the cheese with a reduced-fat cheese.

In a large frying pan, warm ½ teaspoon of the oil over medium heat until hot. Stir in the pepper and sauté 2–3 minutes until the pepper begins to soften. Stir in the spring onions and sauté for 1 minute. Remove from the heat and stir in the coriander and the chillies. Transfer the mixture to a small bowl. Reserve the frying pan to use again.

Place 4 of the corn tortillas on a countertop or chopping board. Sprinkle each tortilla with 1 tablespoon of the cheese, then top each one with one-quarter of the pepper mixture, another ½ tablespoon of the cheese, and then the 4 remaining tortillas.

With a pastry brush, brush the remaining oil over the tops of the tortillas. Place the frying pan over medium heat. Carefully add 2 filled tortillas and cook 2–3 minutes per side until lightly browned. Repeat with the 2 remaining filled tortillas. Cut the quesadillas into quarters, divide the quarters among individual plates, and serve immediately.

NUTRIENT ANALYSIS FOR ONE SERVING

Calories 180	Carbohydrates 27 g	Total Fat 6 g
Protein 6 g	Fibre 3 g	Saturated Fat 2 g
Sodium 144 mg	Sugars 1 g	Monounsaturated Fat 1 g
Cholesterol 9 mg		Polyunsaturated Fat 1 g

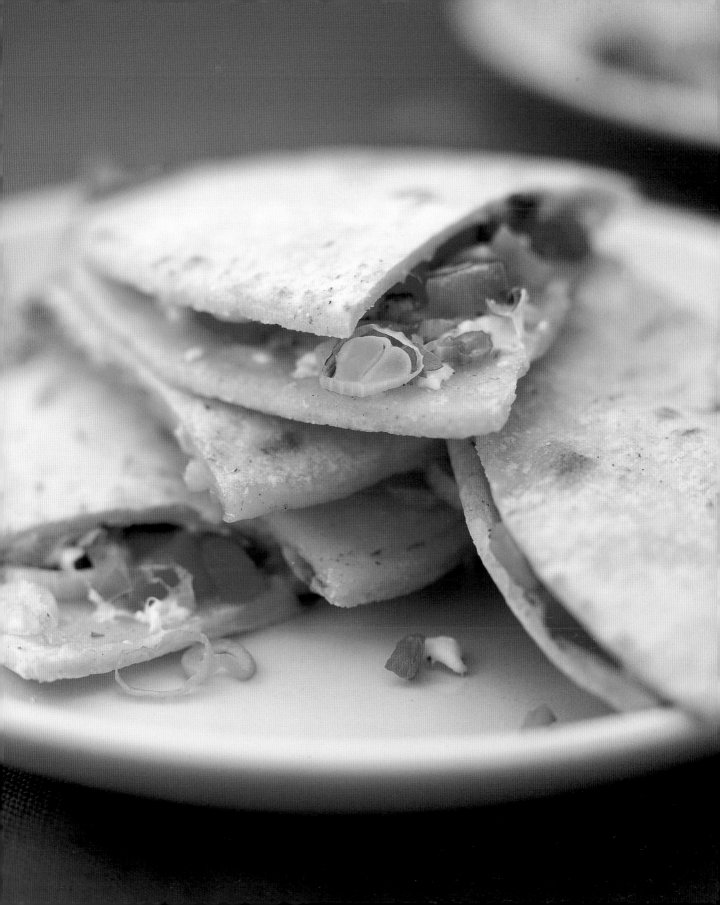

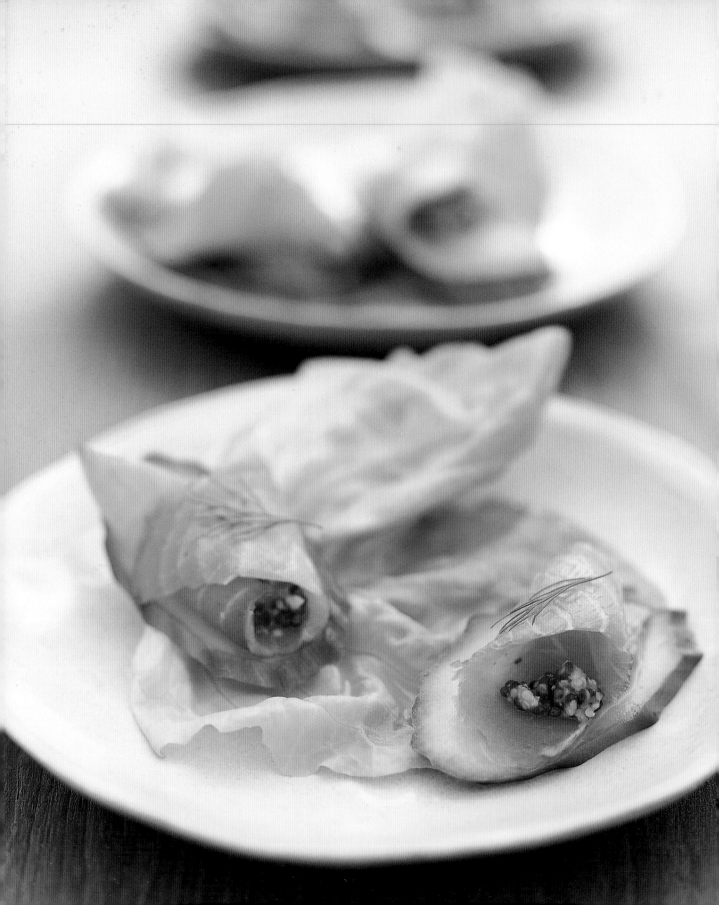

SMOKED SALMON WITH CUCUMBER & DILL

SERVES 4

This elegant starter can be prepared in less than 10 minutes. It features thin slices of heart-healthy salmon flavoured lightly with spicy mustard. Compare brands of packaged cured salmon to find the one with the lowest sodium content.

Place a little mustard on one side of each salmon slice. Arrange a couple of salad leaves on each individual salad plate. Set aside.

Arrange cucumber on the leaves.

For each serving, roll 2 salmon slices and place on top of the cucumber slices and garnish with dill sprigs.

2 teaspoons coarse-grained or Dijon mustard

100 g (4 oz) thinly sliced smoked salmon, cut into 8 pieces

Few salad leaves

8 slices cucumber, sliced diagonally

Few sprigs fresh dill

NUTRIENT ANALYSIS FOR ONE SERVING

Calories 35	**Carbohydrates** 2 g	**Total Fat** 1 g
Protein 6 g	**Fibre** 1 g	**Saturated Fat** 0 g
Sodium 390 mg	**Sugars** 1 g	**Monounsaturated Fat** 0 g
Cholesterol 10 mg		**Polyunsaturated Fat** 0 g

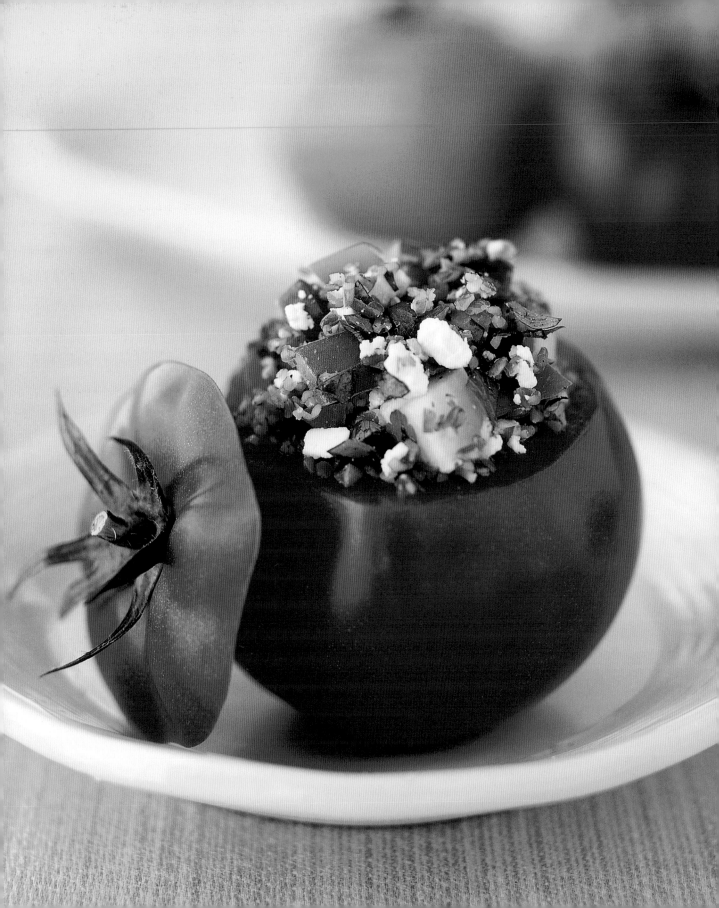

TOMATOES STUFFED WITH CUCUMBER & FETA CHEESE

SERVES 4

Fresh herbs and vegetables tossed with bulgur, a chewy whole grain that's quick and easy to prepare, make a healthy filling for these Mediterranean-style stuffed tomatoes. Substitute cooked brown rice for the prepared bulgur if you like.

In a bowl, combine the bulgur, boiling water, and lemon juice. Let stand for about 30 minutes until most of the liquid has been absorbed. Add the cucumber, red onion, most of the feta cheese, green and red peppers, parsley, and oregano; toss gently to mix.

In a separate small bowl, combine the red wine vinegar, olive oil, pepper, and salt. Whisk until well blended. Drizzle the vinaigrette over the bulgur mixture and toss gently to blend. Cover and refrigerate until ready to use.

Just before serving, cut off the tops of the tomatoes. Reserve the tops. With a spoon or melon baller, scoop out and discard the tomato seeds and ribs.

Remove the bulgur mixture from the refrigerator and, with a spoon, divide the mixture evenly among the scooped-out tomatoes. Sprinkle the remaining feta cheese over the top of the filling and garnish with the tomato tops.

90 g (3½ oz) bulgur

85 ml (2½ fl oz) boiling water

2 tablespoons fresh lemon juice

¼ small cucumber, peeled, seeded, and chopped

1 small red onion, chopped

50 g (2 oz) feta cheese, crumbled

¼ green sweet pepper, seeded and chopped

½ red sweet pepper, seeded and chopped

2 tablespoons chopped fresh parsley

½ tablespoon chopped fresh oregano or 1 teaspoon dried oregano

1 tablespoon red wine vinegar

2½ teaspoons olive oil

¼ teaspoon freshly ground black pepper

⅛ teaspoon salt

4 large red, yellow, or orange tomatoes, about 700 g (1½ lb) total weight

NUTRIENT ANALYSIS FOR ONE SERVING

Calories 156	**Carbohydrates** 24 g	**Total Fat** 6 g
Protein 8 g	**Fibre** 6 g	**Saturated Fat** 2 g
Sodium 198 mg	**Sugars** 6 g	**Monounsaturated Fat** 3 g
Cholesterol 8 mg		**Polyunsaturated Fat** 1 g

VEGETABLE PLATTER WITH HUMMUS DIP

150 g (5 oz) broccoli florets

150 g (5 oz) cauliflower florets

2 large cloves garlic, chopped

One 400-g (14-oz) tin chickpeas, rinsed and drained

175 g (6 oz) reduced-fat silken tofu, cut into 1-cm (½-in) cubes

3 tablespoons fresh lemon juice

1 tablespoon chopped fresh mint or 1 teaspoon dried mint, plus several fresh mint sprigs (optional)

2 teaspoons olive oil

1 teaspoon dark sesame oil

¼–½ teaspoon chilli flakes

¼ teaspoon salt

2 red or yellow sweet peppers, or 1 of each, cut into large chunks

150 g (5 oz) baby carrots

The vegetables in this appetizer taste delicious with hummus, a Middle Eastern dip made of chickpeas, sesame, lemon, and garlic. You can substitute 100 g (4 oz) dried chickpeas for the tinned beans. (For tips on cooking dried beans, see page 135.)

Bring a large saucepan three-quarters full of water to a boil. Add the broccoli and cauliflower and return to a boil. Cook about 1 minute until the vegetables are tender-crisp. Drain the vegetables and then plunge them into a bowl of ice water to stop the cooking. Drain again and set aside.

In a food processor or blender, process the chickpeas and garlic until finely chopped. Add the tofu, lemon juice, chopped mint, 1 teaspoon of the olive oil, the sesame oil, chilli flakes, and salt and process until smooth. Transfer the hummus to a serving bowl and drizzle with the remaining olive oil.

To serve, arrange the broccoli, cauliflower, peppers, and carrots on a serving platter and garnish with the mint sprigs, if desired. Place the bowl of hummus alongside as a dip for the vegetables.

NUTRIENT ANALYSIS FOR ONE SERVING

Calories 138	**Carbohydrates** 21 g	**Total Fat** 4 g
Protein 7 g	**Fibre** 6 g	**Saturated Fat** 1 g
Sodium 140 mg	**Sugars** 4 g	**Monounsaturated Fat** 2 g
Cholesterol 0 mg		**Polyunsaturated Fat** 1 g

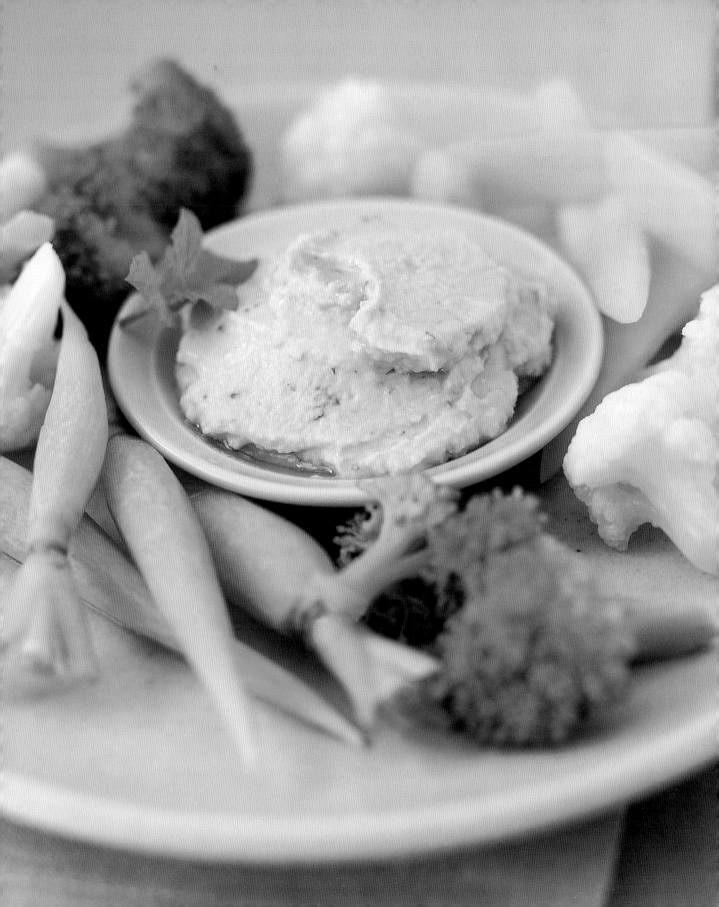

HOT & SOUR SOUP

DIABETIC EXCHANGES

½ starch	0 fruit	0 milk
½ vegetable	1 protein	½ fat

SERVES 6

175 g (6 oz) reduced-fat, extra-firm tofu, cut int 1-cm (½-in) cubes

3 tablespoons low-sodium soy sauce

2 teaspoons dark sesame oil

175 g (6 oz) fresh shiitake mushrooms, brushed clean, stemmed, and sliced

1.2 l (2 pt) fat-free, no-salt-added chicken stock

100 g (4 oz) mangetout, trimmed and cut lengthwise into thin strips

3 tablespoons rice vinegar

½ teaspoon chilli flakes or 1 teaspoon hot chilli oil

2 tablespoons cornflour

2 tablespoons water

3 tablespoons chopped fresh coriander or thinly sliced spring onion

This crowd-pleasing soup is remarkably easy to prepare and goes from cooker to table in less than 15 minutes. Fresh shiitake mushrooms give the soup a delicate flavour, but use readily available button mushrooms as a delicious alternative.

Toss the tofu with the soy sauce and set aside.

In a large saucepan, heat the sesame oil over medium heat until hot. Add the mushrooms and cook about 5 minutes, stirring occasionally, until the mushrooms are tender. Add the stock, mangetout, vinegar, and chilli flakes to the saucepan with the mushrooms. Bring to a boil over high heat. Reduce the heat to low and simmer, uncovered, for 5 minutes.

Combine the cornflour and water and stir to mix well. Add the cornflour mixture to the soup and simmer for about 1 minute until the soup is thickened. Add the tofu mixture, return to a simmer, and cook for about 1 minute until heated through. Stir in the coriander and serve.

NUTRIENT ANALYSIS FOR ONE SERVING

Calories 82	**Carbohydrates** 6 g	**Total Fat** 2 g
Protein 8 g	**Fibre** 1 g	**Saturated Fat** 0 g
Sodium 461 mg	**Sugars** 1 g	**Monounsaturated Fat** 1 g
Cholesterol 0 mg		**Polyunsaturated Fat** 1 g

MUSHROOM BARLEY SOUP

CARB COUNT 16g

DIABETIC EXCHANGES
| ½ starch | 0 fruit | 0 milk |
| 1½ vegetable | 1 protein | ½ fat |

SERVES 6

Fresh and dried mushrooms contribute subtle woodsy flavours and aromas to this satisfying soup. Find dried mushrooms in the international section of your supermarket. Use kitchen scissors to snip them into small pieces before soaking.

In a small heatproof glass measuring cup or bowl, combine the dried porcini and boiling water. Let stand for 20 minutes. Remove the porcini with a slotted spoon and set aside. Line a fine-mesh sieve with a paper coffee filter or cheesecloth and strain the porcini soaking liquid to remove the grit; reserve the liquid.

While the porcini are soaking, in a large saucepan, heat the olive oil over medium-high heat. Add the shallots and cook for 3 minutes, stirring occasionally, until softened. Add the sliced fresh mushrooms and cook for 3 minutes, stirring occasionally, until lightly browned. Add the stock, barley, and carrots and bring to a simmer. Reduce the heat to low. Add the porcini, reserved porcini soaking liquid, thyme, bay leaf, salt, and pepper. Simmer about 25 minutes, uncovered, stirring occasionally, until the barley is tender. Remove the bay leaf and serve.

7 g (¼ oz) snipped or chopped dried porcini mushrooms

250 ml (8 fl oz) boiling water

2 teaspoons olive oil

4 shallots, chopped

225 g (8 oz) fresh chestnut or button mushrooms, sliced, or sliced mixed fresh mushrooms, such as oyster, chestnut, and shiitake

1.5 l (2½ pt) fat-free, no-salt-added beef stock

50 g (2 oz) quick-cooking pearl barley

2 small carrots, thinly sliced

1 tablespoon chopped fresh thyme or 1 teaspoon dried thyme

1 bay leaf

¾ teaspoon salt

¼ teaspoon freshly ground black pepper

NUTRIENT ANALYSIS FOR ONE SERVING

Calories 111	**Carbohydrates** 16 g	**Total Fat** 2 g
Protein 9 g	**Fibre** 3 g	**Saturated Fat** 0 g
Sodium 478 mg	**Sugars** 2 g	**Monounsaturated Fat** 1 g
Cholesterol 0 mg		**Polyunsaturated Fat** 0 g

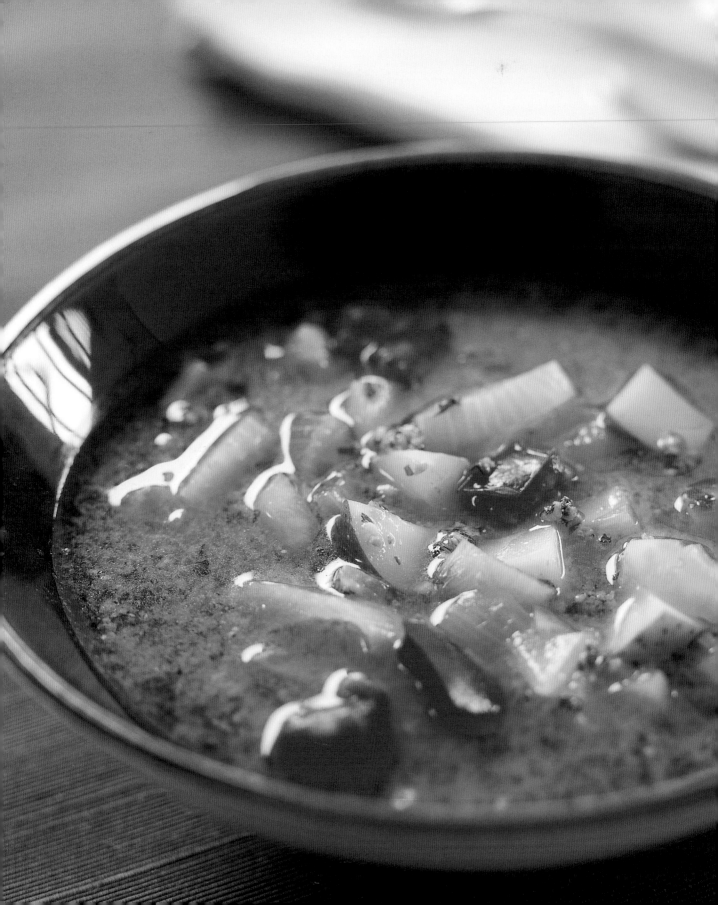

VEGETABLE SOUP WITH BASIL & PINE NUTS

DIABETIC EXCHANGES

| ½ starch | 0 fruit | 0 milk |
| 2 vegetable | ½ protein | ½ fat |

SERVES 6

This simple dish is based on a classic vegetable stew known as *soupe au pistou* in France. It gets a burst of flavour from fresh basil. If fresh fennel isn't available, use two chopped celery stalks or 225 g (8 oz) green beans, trimmed and cut into pieces.

Put the pine nuts in a small, dry non-stick frying pan over medium-high heat. Cook 1–2 minutes, stirring often, until lightly toasted. Set aside.

In a large saucepan, heat the olive oil over medium-high heat. Add the onion, fennel, and garlic and sauté about 5 minutes, until fragrant. Stir in the potatoes and stock. Cover and bring to a simmer over high heat. Reduce the heat to low and simmer, covered, for 15–20 minutes, until the vegetables are just tender. Stir in the chopped tomato, salt, and pepper and continue to simmer for about 2 minutes, until the tomato is softened.

While the soup is simmering, in a food processor or blender, combine the basil leaves and toasted pine nuts. Process until very finely chopped. Stir the mixture into the soup and ladle the soup into individual bowls.

3 tablespoons pine nuts

1 teaspoon olive oil

1 onion, chopped

1 fennel bulb, chopped

3 cloves garlic, crushed

225 g (8 oz) chopped potatoes, cut into 1-cm (½-in) pieces

1 l (1¾ pt) fat-free, no-salt-added vegetable or chicken stock

1 large tomato, seeded and chopped

¼ teaspoon salt

¼ teaspoon freshly ground black pepper

15 g (½ oz) packed fresh basil leaves

NUTRIENT ANALYSIS FOR ONE SERVING

Calories 109	Carbohydrates 17 g	Total Fat 3 g
Protein 4 g	Fibre 4 g	Saturated Fat 0 g
Sodium 430 mg	Sugars 5 g	Monounsaturated Fat 1 g
Cholesterol 0 mg		Polyunsaturated Fat 1 g

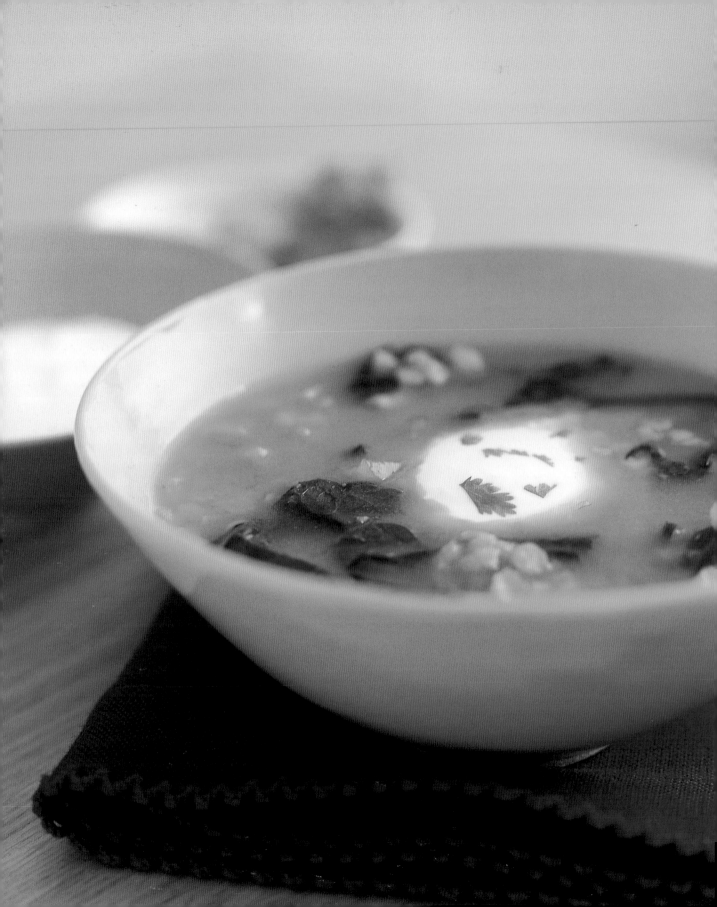

RED LENTIL SOUP

SERVES 6

CARB COUNT 23g

DIABETIC EXCHANGES

| 1 starch | 0 fruit | 0 milk |
| ½ vegetable | 1 protein | ½ fat |

Quick-cooking red lentils have a mild flavour that pairs nicely with curry powder. If you can't find Madras curry, use regular curry powder and add a pinch of cayenne. Brown lentils may be substituted; simmer the soup 8 to 10 minutes longer.

In a large saucepan, heat the oil over medium heat. Add the onion and garlic and cook about 5 minutes, stirring occasionally, until soft and fragrant. Sprinkle the curry powder and cardamom over the onion mixture and cook, stirring, for 1 minute longer.

Add the stock, lentils, and salt and bring to a boil over high heat. Reduce the heat to low and simmer 20–25 minutes, uncovered, stirring occasionally, until the lentils are tender. Stir in the Swiss chard and cook for about 5 minutes, stirring once, until the chard is tender. Ladle into individual shallow bowls and top with the yoghurt and coriander.

2 teaspoons olive oil or sunflower oil

1 onion, chopped

4 cloves garlic, crushed

2 teaspoons Madras or hot curry powder

½ teaspoon ground cardamom

1.2 l (2 pt) fat-free, no-salt-added chicken or vegetable stock

150 g (5 oz) dried red lentils

½ teaspoon salt

75 g (3 oz) coarsely chopped Swiss chard or kale

4 tablespoons low-fat plain yoghurt

4 tablespoons chopped fresh coriander

NUTRIENT ANALYSIS FOR ONE SERVING

Calories 164	Carbohydrates 23 g	Total Fat 2 g
Protein 10 g	Fibre 6 g	Saturated Fat 0 g
Sodium 490 mg	Sugars 4 g	Monounsaturated Fat 1 g
Cholesterol 1 mg		Polyunsaturated Fat 0 g

CHICKEN SOUP WITH ROSEMARY & GARLIC

DIABETIC EXCHANGES

1 starch	0 fruit	0 milk
0 vegetable	2½ protein	½ fat

SERVES 6

2 teaspoons olive oil

4 cloves garlic, crushed

225 g (8 oz) skinless, boneless chicken breasts, cut into 1-cm (½-in) chunks

2 courgettes, cut into 1-cm (½-in) chunks

1 tablespoon chopped fresh rosemary or 1 teaspoon dried rosemary

½ teaspoon salt

¼ teaspoon freshly ground black pepper

1 l (1¾ pt) fat-free, no-salt-added chicken stock

6 slices wholemeal baguette, 1-cm (½-in) thick, toasted

6 tablespoons grated Parmesan or Romano cheese

Rich with the irresistible flavours of Tuscany—olive oil, garlic, rosemary, and a bit of freshly grated cheese—this soup is hearty enough to serve as a main course or as a substantial first course in a dinner with a light pasta dish and a salad.

In a saucepan, heat the olive oil over medium heat. Add the garlic and sauté for 2 minutes. Add the chicken, courgettes, rosemary, salt, and pepper and sauté for 2 minutes. Add the stock and bring to a simmer over high heat. Reduce the heat to low and simmer, uncovered, about 8 minutes, until the chicken is cooked through and the courgettes are tender.

Ladle the soup into individual bowls and top each serving with a slice of toasted baguette and 1 tablespoon of the cheese.

NUTRIENT ANALYSIS FOR ONE SERVING

Calories 177	Carbohydrates 15 g	Total Fat 5 g
Protein 18 g	**Fibre** 3 g	**Saturated Fat** 2 g
Sodium 491 mg	**Sugars** 2 g	**Monounsaturated Fat** 2 g
Cholesterol 28 mg		**Polyunsaturated Fat** 1 g

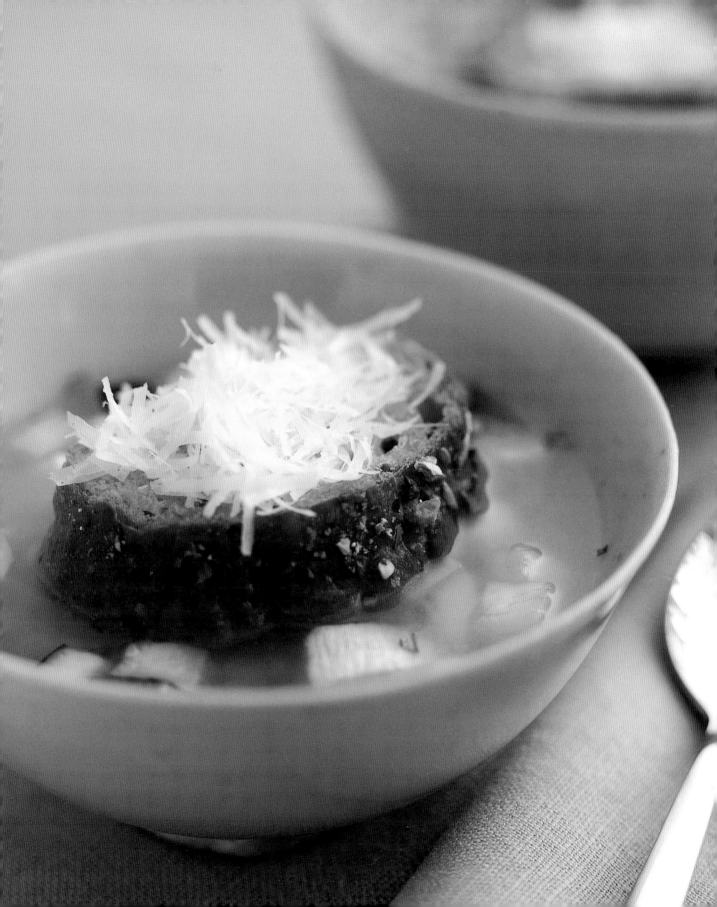

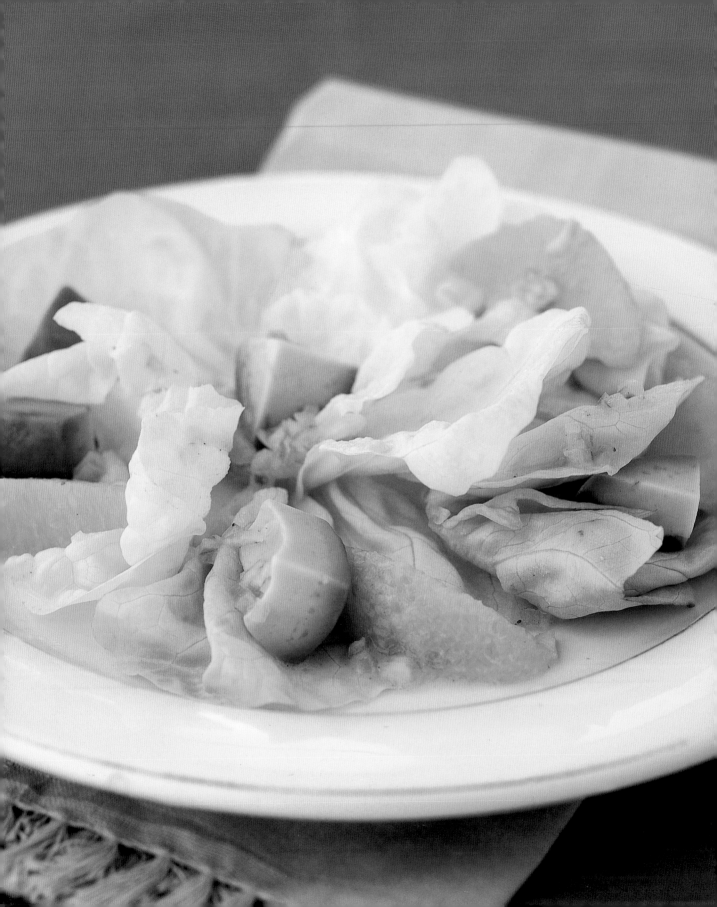

LETTUCE SALAD WITH ORANGE & AVOCADO

CARB COUNT **17**g

DIABETIC EXCHANGES

| 0 starch | 1 fruit | 0 milk |
| ½ vegetable | 0 protein | 1 fat |

SERVES 4

In this classic tossed salad, chunks of creamy, mild avocado contrast deliciously with the intense sweet-and-sour tang of fresh orange. You can use 1 large orange instead of small navel oranges, and cut the peeled segments in half.

In a large bowl, combine the lettuce, avocado, and orange segments.

In a small bowl, combine the orange juice, shallots, mustard, honey, salt, and pepper and stir to mix well.

Pour the orange juice mixture over the lettuce mixture and toss well. Transfer to individual plates and serve immediately.

1 small round lettuce, torn into pieces

½ ripe avocado, stoned, peeled, and cut into 2-cm (¾-in) chunks

2 small navel oranges, peeled and separated into segments

60 ml (2 fl oz) orange juice

1 tablespoon shallots, chopped

2 teaspoons Dijon mustard

½ teaspoon runny honey

¼ teaspoon salt

¼ teaspoon freshly ground black pepper

NUTRIENT ANALYSIS FOR ONE SERVING

Calories 103	**Carbohydrates** 17 g	**Total Fat** 4 g
Protein 3 g	**Fibre** 5 g	**Saturated Fat** 1 g
Sodium 159 mg	**Sugars** 11 g	**Monounsaturated Fat** 2 g
Cholesterol 0 mg		**Polyunsaturated Fat** 1 g

9g

ASPARAGUS WITH SHALLOTS & BLUE CHEESE

DIABETIC EXCHANGES

0 starch	0 fruit	0 milk
1 vegetable	½ protein	½ fat

SERVES 4

½ wholemeal muffin, torn into chunks

1 teaspoon walnut oil or olive oil

1 shallot, chopped

16 asparagus spears, trimmed

3 tablespoons fat-free, no-salt-added chicken stock

1 tablespoon white wine vinegar or sherry vinegar

⅛ teaspoon salt

¼ teaspoon freshly ground black pepper

4 large leaves lollo rosso lettuce or other salad leaves

15 g (½ oz) Gorgonzola or other blue cheese, crumbled

Served at room temperature, this salad of asparagus and fresh greens goes well with a dish such as Seared Sirloin with Sweet Potato Ragout (page 73). The salad and dressing can be made up to 2 hours ahead; refrigerate them separately until serving.

Place the muffin chunks in a food processor or blender and process to coarse crumbs. Heat the oil in a large non-stick frying pan over high heat. Add the shallot and sauté about 3 minutes, stirring occasionally, until tender. Add the muffin crumbs and continue cooking 2–3 minutes, stirring constantly, until the shallots and crumbs are crisp. Remove from the heat and let stand while preparing the salad.

In a large pot fitted with a steamer basket, bring 2.5 cm (1 in) of water to a boil. Add the asparagus, cover, and steam about 4 minutes, until the asparagus is tender-crisp. Drain the asparagus, then plunge the spears into a bowl of ice water to stop the cooking. Drain again and set aside.

In a small bowl, combine the stock, vinegar, salt, and pepper and mix well.

Place 1 lettuce leaf on each plate. Arrange 4 asparagus spears on each lettuce leaf and top with the crumb mixture and cheese. Stir the dressing and drizzle it evenly over the salads.

NUTRIENT ANALYSIS FOR ONE SERVING

Calories 64	Carbohydrates 9 g	Total Fat 2 g
Protein 4 g	Fibre 2 g	Saturated Fat 1 g
Sodium 186 mg	Sugars 2 g	Monounsaturated Fat 0 g
Cholesterol 2 mg		Polyunsaturated Fat 1 g

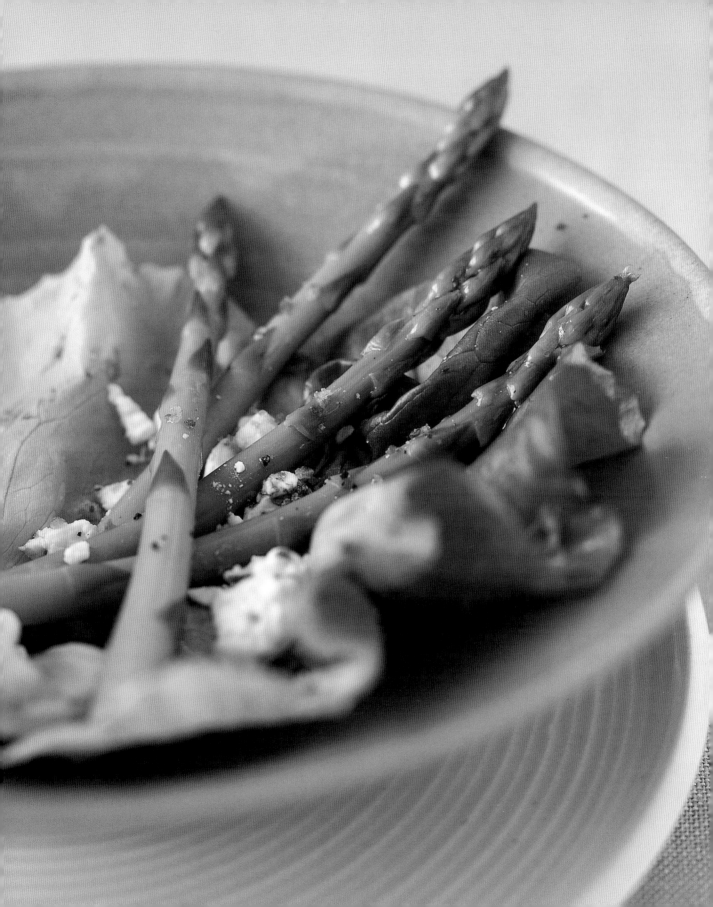

30g

BULGUR SALAD WITH ROCKET & OLIVES

SERVES 4

200 g (7 oz) bulgur

375 ml (12 fl oz) boiling water

85 ml (2½ fl oz) fat-free, no-salt-added chicken or vegetable stock

2 tablespoons fresh lemon juice

1 tablespoon olive oil

¼ teaspoon freshly ground black pepper

1 large tomato or 2 plum tomatoes, seeded and chopped

25 g (1 oz) packed coarsely chopped rocket or watercress

25 g (1 oz) sliced pitted black olives

2 tablespoons chopped fresh mint

Traditionally made with parsley, the Mediterranean salad called tabbouleh takes on a hint of Italy when made instead with rocket, a mustard-family green. Chop the vegetables while the bulgur soaks and serve the salad at room temperature.

Place the bulgur in a large, heatproof bowl and add the boiling water. Let stand about 25 minutes until the bulgur is tender and the water is completely absorbed.

Add the stock, lemon juice, olive oil, pepper, tomato, rocket, olives, and mint. Toss gently just until the ingredients are evenly distributed. Serve at room temperature, or cover and refrigerate for up to 2 hours.

NUTRIENT ANALYSIS FOR ONE SERVING

Calories 188	**Carbohydrates** 30 g	**Total Fat** 6 g
Protein 5 g	**Fibre** 7 g	**Saturated Fat** 1 g
Sodium 181 mg	**Sugars** 2 g	**Monounsaturated Fat** 4 g
Cholesterol 0 mg		**Polyunsaturated Fat** 1 g

CHOPPED SALAD WITH LIME-AVOCADO DRESSING

CARB COUNT 28g

DIABETIC EXCHANGES

| ½ starch | 0 fruit | 0 milk |
| 1½ vegetable | 0 protein | 1 fat |

SERVES 4

Compatible ingredients including tomatoes, fresh sweetcorn, cumin, chillies, and freshly toasted tortilla chips give this salad an appealing Mexican flavour. A bit of chicken stock lightens the dressing. Serve alongside roasted or grilled fish.

Preheat the oven to 200°C (400°F). Stack the tortillas and cut them into quarters to form 16 wedges. Arrange the wedges in a single layer on a baking sheet. Bake 10–12 minutes, until golden brown and crisp. Transfer the toasted tortilla wedges to a plate; set aside.

While the tortillas are toasting, line each individual plate with 2 lettuce leaves, cut or torn in half, if necessary, to fit. In a large bowl, combine the chopped lettuce, tomato, carrot, and sweetcorn. In a food processor or blender, combine the avocado, chilli, stock, lime juice, sunflower oil, cumin, and salt and process until puréed. Add the dressing to the chopped lettuce mixture and toss to coat. Divide the salad among the lettuce-lined plates. Garnish with the tortilla chips.

- 4 corn tortillas, 15 cm (6 in) in diameter
- 1 head cos (romaine lettuce), 8 outer leaves left whole, remaining inner leaves coarsely chopped
- 1 large tomato, chopped
- 1 large carrot, cut into julienne or coarsely grated
- 175 g (6 oz) fresh or frozen sweetcorn kernels, thawed
- ½ large avocado, stoned, peeled, and diced
- 1 red or green chilli, seeded and chopped
- 2 tablespoons fat-free, no-salt-added chicken or vegetable stock
- 1 tablespoon fresh lime juice
- 1 teaspoon sunflower oil
- ½ teaspoon ground cumin
- ¼ teaspoon salt

NUTRIENT ANALYSIS FOR ONE SERVING

Calories 161	**Carbohydrates** 28 g	**Total Fat** 5 g
Protein 5 g	**Fibre** 6 g	**Saturated Fat** 1 g
Sodium 167 mg	**Sugars** 3 g	**Monounsaturated Fat** 3 g
Cholesterol 0 mg		**Polyunsaturated Fat** 1 g

BEETROOT & SPINACH SALAD

SERVES 4

4 beetroot, about 575 g (1¼ lb) total weight

125 ml (4 fl oz) water

100 g (4 oz) packed baby spinach or torn spinach leaves

3 tablespoons fat-free, no-salt-added chicken or vegetable stock

2½ tablespoons balsamic vinegar

1 teaspoon olive oil

1 tablespoon Dijon mustard

½ teaspoon runny honey

¼ teaspoon freshly ground black pepper

⅛ teaspoon salt

2 tablespoons dry-roasted, unsalted pistachios or toasted pine nuts (page 138)

Very colourful to begin with, this light salad looks even bolder and brighter when made with a mixture of red and golden beetroot. Look for unusual beet varieties at farmers' markets.

Preheat the oven to 190°C (375°F).

Trim off the beet greens and reserve for another use. Rinse the beetroot well and arrange them, unpeeled, in a single layer in a shallow baking dish. Add the water and cover the dish with aluminium foil. Roast 35–45 minutes until the beets are tender.

Transfer the roasted beetroot to a colander and rinse with cold water. Let stand until cool enough to handle. With a small sharp knife, peel the beetroot and cut them into wedges.

Combine the beetroot slices and spinach in a large bowl. In a separate bowl, combine the stock, vinegar, olive oil, mustard, honey, pepper, and salt and stir to mix well. Add the stock-vinegar mixture to the spinach-beet mixture and toss well to coat. Transfer to individual plates and top with the pistachio nuts.

NUTRIENT ANALYSIS FOR ONE SERVING

Calories 101	Carbohydrates 14 g	Total Fat 4 g
Protein 4 g	Fibre 3 g	Saturated Fat 1 g
Sodium 191 mg	Sugars 10 g	Monounsaturated Fat 2 g
Cholesterol 0 mg		Polyunsaturated Fat 1 g

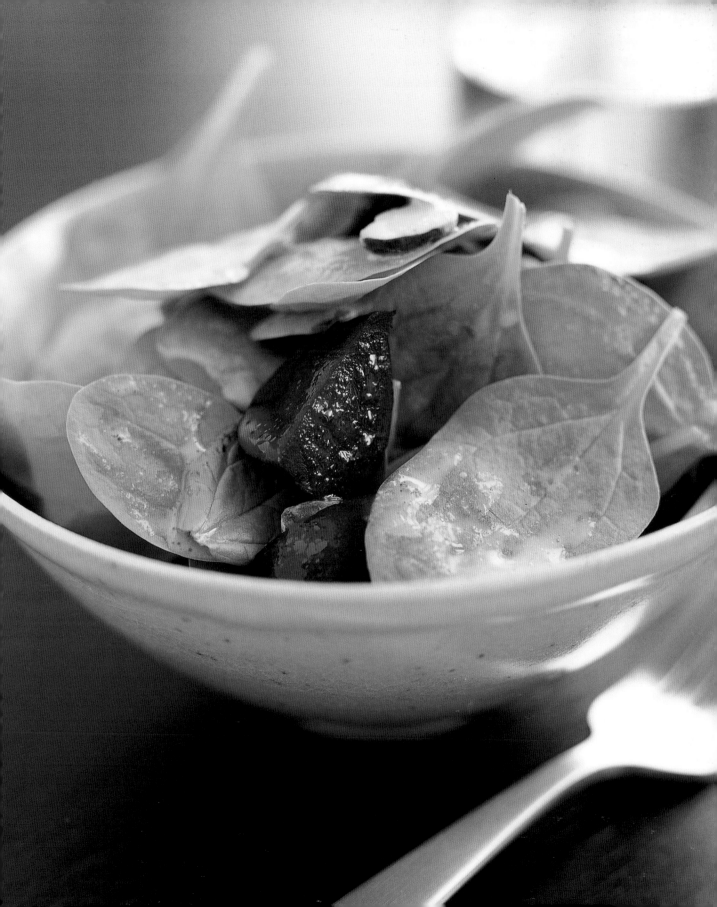

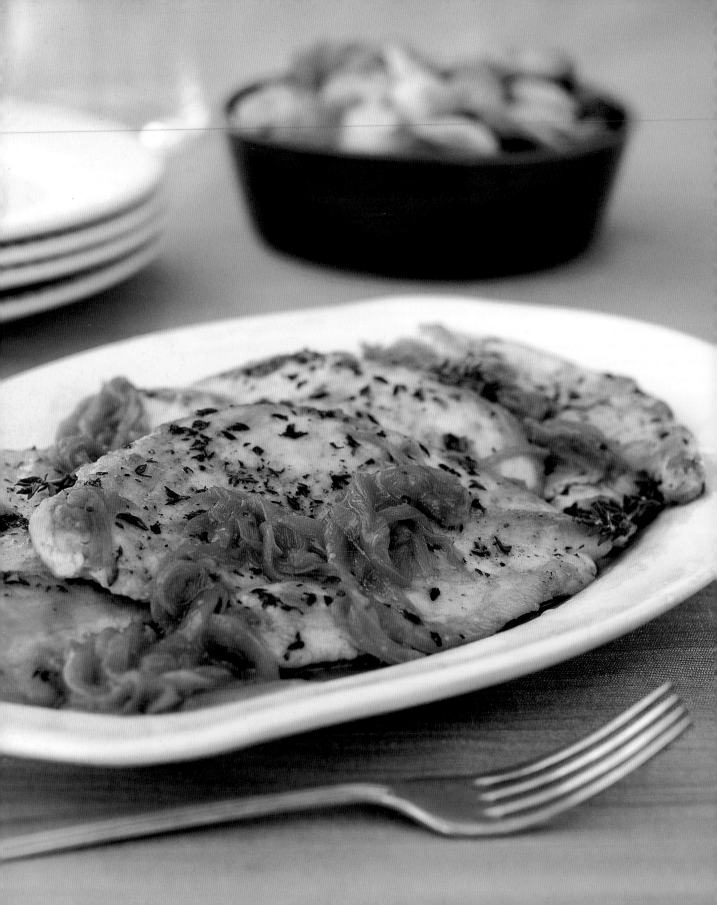

MAIN DISHES

Chicken with Caramelized Onions, 64

OVEN-BARBECUED SALMON

SERVES 4

125 ml (4 fl oz) orange juice

2 tablespoons fresh lemon juice

4 skinless salmon fillets, each 150 g (5 oz) and about 3 cm (1¼ in) thick

1 tablespoon firmly packed light brown sugar

1 tablespoon paprika

½ teaspoon salt

½ teaspoon garlic powder

½ teaspoon onion powder

½ teaspoon ground coriander

¼ teaspoon ground cinnamon

¼ teaspoon cayenne pepper

⅛ teaspoon ground cumin

½ teaspoon sunflower oil

Tangy citrus juices blended with several spices make a complex, barbecue-style rub that complements the rich flavour of baked salmon. Although the list of spices is long, it takes just a minute or two to combine the ingredients for this satisfying dish.

In a large shallow non-metallic container or lock-top plastic bag, combine the orange and lemon juices. Add the salmon fillets, turn to coat, cover or seal the container, and refrigerate for 30 minutes.

In a small bowl, combine the brown sugar, paprika, salt, garlic powder, onion powder, coriander, cinnamon, cayenne, and cumin.

Preheat the oven to 200°C (400°F).

Lightly coat the bottom of a shallow baking dish with the sunflower oil. Remove the fish from the marinade and pat dry with paper towels. Discard the marinade. Place the fish in the oiled baking dish. Rub the top and sides of the fish with the spice mixture. Bake 10–12 minutes until the fish is opaque throughout when tested in the centre with the tip of a knife. Transfer the baked fillets to warmed individual plates and serve immediately.

NUTRIENT ANALYSIS FOR ONE SERVING

Calories 228	Carbohydrates 5 g	Total Fat 10 g
Protein 29 g	Fibre 1 g	Saturated Fat 1 g
Sodium 358 mg	Sugars 3 g	Monounsaturated Fat 3 g
Cholesterol 78 mg		Polyunsaturated Fat 4 g

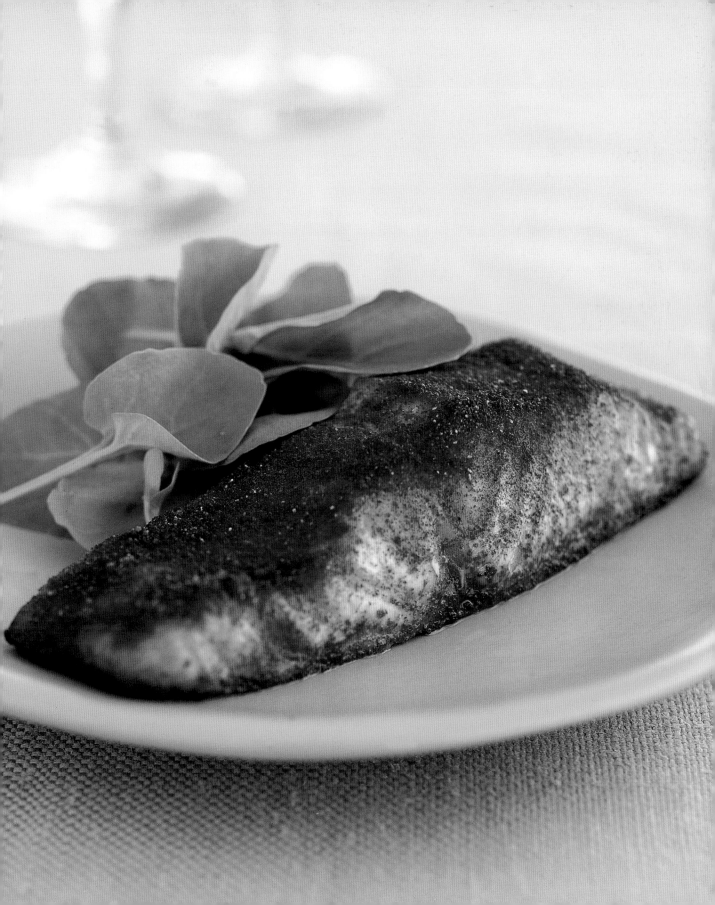

COD BAKED IN SPINACH LEAVES

SERVES 4

10 large basil leaves

15 g (½ oz) coarsely chopped spinach

2 tablespoons coarsely chopped parsley

1 tablespoon coarsely chopped almonds

1 clove garlic, crushed

2 teaspoons olive oil or sunflower oil

2 teaspoons lemon juice

¼ teaspoon salt

¼ teaspoon freshly ground black pepper

4 cod or turbot fillets, each 150 g (5 oz) and about 3 cm (1¼ in) thick

20 large spinach leaves, each about 12 x 15 cm (5 x 6 in), tough stems removed

1 lemon, sliced into 12 thin circles

Any firm, white-fleshed fish works well in this elegant dish. Fillets are topped with a simple basil-almond pesto, wrapped in spinach leaves, and baked. A store-bought pesto can stand in for home-made, but it will likely be higher in fat and calories.

Preheat the oven to 190°C (375°F).

In a small food processor or blender, combine the basil, chopped spinach, parsley, almonds, garlic, oil, lemon juice, and ⅛ teaspoon of the salt. Pulse to blend.

Sprinkle the remaining salt and the pepper on the fish. Top each fillet with a dollop of pesto.

Place 5 spinach leaves on a paper towel and microwave 15 seconds on high or until the spinach wilts but is still bright green; let cool slightly. On a chopping board or flat surface, arrange 3 wilted spinach leaves, overlapping them slightly. Place a pesto-topped fish fillet in the centre of the leaves. Top with 2 more spinach leaves, making sure to cover the fish completely. Using your fingers, press the leaves together to seal. Repeat the procedure with the remaining spinach leaves and fish. Place 3 lemon slices across the top of each spinach-wrapped fillet, overlapping them slightly.

Place the wrapped fillets on a baking sheet lined with parchment paper or aluminium foil. Bake for about 15 minutes until the fish is firm to the touch. Serve immediately.

NUTRIENT ANALYSIS FOR ONE SERVING

Calories 186	**Carbohydrates** 3 g	**Total Fat** 6 g
Protein 30 g	**Fibre** 2 g	**Saturated Fat** 1 g
Sodium 265 mg	**Sugars** 0 g	**Monounsaturated Fat** 3 g
Cholesterol 52 mg		**Polyunsaturated Fat** 1 g

POLENTA-CRUSTED HADDOCK FILLETS

DIABETIC EXCHANGES

½ starch	0 fruit	0 milk
0 vegetable	4½ protein	1 fat

SERVES 4

Dusted with spiced polenta and browned, the haddock in this recipe cooks up crisp outside and tender inside. Other thin fillets of fish, such as cod, plaice, or pollack, also work well in this dish. Try it paired with Soya Bean Succotash (page 102).

In a shallow dish, combine the polenta, parsley, paprika, salt, garlic powder, onion flakes, and cayenne. Stir to blend.

In another shallow dish, combine the egg whites and water, and whisk to blend. Dip the fish in the egg whites, then dredge in the polenta mixture to coat.

In a large non-stick frying pan, heat the oil over medium-high heat. Add the fish and cook, 2–3 minutes per side, turning once, until the fish is opaque throughout when tested in the centre with a tip of a knife and the coating is lightly browned.

4 tablespoons polenta

2 tablespoons chopped fresh parsley

1 teaspoon paprika

¼ teaspoon salt

½ teaspoon garlic powder

½ teaspoon dried onion flakes

⅛ teaspoon cayenne pepper

2 egg whites, lightly beaten

1 tablespoon water

4 skinless haddock fillets, each 150 g (5 oz) and about 1 cm (½ in) thick

1½ tablespoons olive oil or sunflower oil

NUTRIENT ANALYSIS FOR ONE SERVING

Calories 231	**Carbohydrates** 8 g	**Total Fat** 7 g
Protein 32 g	**Fibre** 1 g	**Saturated Fat** 1 g
Sodium 265 mg	**Sugars** 0 g	**Monounsaturated Fat** 3 g
Cholesterol 52 mg		**Polyunsaturated Fat** 2 g

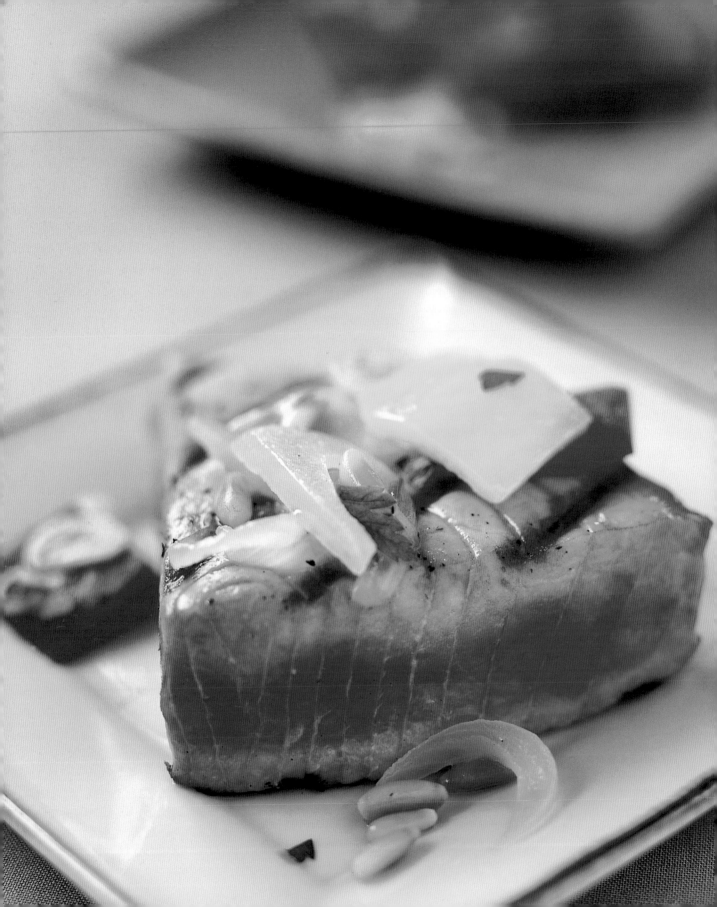

GRILLED TUNA WITH PEPPER & ONION SALSA

CARB COUNT

4 g

DIABETIC EXCHANGES

| 0 starch | 0 fruit | 0 milk |
| 1 vegetable | 5 protein | 1 fat |

SERVES 4

Fresh tuna is most likely to stay moist and tender during grilling when it's first brushed lightly with oil. Prepare and chill the salsa ahead of time if you like, but for the best flavour bring it to room temperature before serving.

Put the pine nuts in a small, dry non-stick frying pan over medium-high heat. Cook 3–5 minutes, stirring often, until lightly toasted. Set aside.

In a large frying pan, heat 2 teaspoons of the olive oil over medium heat. Add the onion and sauté about 4 minutes until it begins to soften. Add the garlic and sauté for 1 minute. Stir in the yellow and red peppers, water, and ¼ teaspoon of the salt. Simmer gently about 10–12 minutes until the liquid evaporates and the peppers are tender-crisp. Remove from the heat and stir in the parsley, pine nuts, vinegar, and a little pepper. Keep warm or let cool to room temperature.

Rub the tuna steaks with the remaining oil. Sprinkle with the remaining salt and the pepper. Cook on a ridged griddle pan, barbecue, or under a preheated grill, for 3–4 minutes per side, until the fish is opaque throughout when tested with the tip of a knife and shows only a small amount of pink in the centre. Transfer to warmed individual plates and serve topped with the salsa.

1 tablespoon pine nuts

3 teaspoons olive oil

¼ onion, sliced

2 cloves garlic, thinly sliced

½ yellow sweet pepper, cut into 2.5-cm (1-in) chunks

½ red sweet pepper, cut into 2.5-cm (1-in) chunks

125 ml (4 fl oz) water

½ teaspoon salt

2 tablespoons chopped fresh parsley

½ teaspoon sherry vinegar or red wine vinegar

¼ teaspoon freshly ground black pepper

4 tuna steaks, each 150 g (5 oz) and about 3 cm (1½ in) thick

NUTRIENT ANALYSIS FOR ONE SERVING

Calories 219	**Carbohydrates** 4 g	**Total Fat** 7 g
Protein 34 g	**Fibre** 1 g	**Saturated Fat** 1 g
Sodium 348 mg	**Sugars** 2 g	**Monounsaturated Fat** 4 g
Cholesterol 64 mg		**Polyunsaturated Fat** 1 g

TERIYAKI SCALLOPS

SERVES 4

175 ml (6 fl oz) pineapple juice

85 ml (2½ fl oz) mirin or rice wine vinegar

2 tablespoons low-sodium soy sauce

2 teaspoons dark sesame oil

1 teaspoon fresh ginger, peeled and grated

1 clove garlic, crushed

16 large scallops, about 575 g (1¼ lb) total weight

1 teaspoon sunflower oil

A home-made teriyaki sauce – low-sodium soy sauce seasoned with pineapple, sesame, ginger, and mirin – preserves the natural sweetness of the scallops in this dish. Mirin is a sweet rice wine found with Asian foods in most supermarkets.

In a glass measuring cup or small bowl, combine the pineapple juice, mirin, soy sauce, sesame oil, ginger, and garlic. Whisk to blend.

Pour half of the pineapple-juice mixture into a small saucepan over medium-high heat and bring to a boil. Reduce the heat to medium and simmer gently, for 20–25 minutes, until the mixture is reduced to a syrup. (Watch to make sure the mixture doesn't burn.)

Place the scallops in a bowl with the remaining half of the pineapple juice mixture. Let marinate for 15 minutes.

While the scallops are marinating, preheat a grill to medium-high. Position the cooking rack 10–15 cm (4–6 in) from the heat source. (Alternatively, the scallops can be cooked without skewers on a hot ridged griddle pan.)

Drain the scallops and discard the marinade. Thread the scallops on metal or wooden skewers, and brush with the sunflower oil. (If you use wooden skewers, soak them in water ahead of time for about 30 minutes so they don't burn.) Grill the scallops for 4–6 minutes, turning frequently, until opaque throughout when tested in the centre with the tip of a knife. Brush the cooked scallops with the pineapple syrup and serve immediately.

NUTRIENT ANALYSIS FOR ONE SERVING

Calories 222	Carbohydrates 14 g	Total Fat 5 g
Protein 25 g	Fibre 0 g	Saturated Fat 1 g
Sodium 497 mg	Sugars 9 g	Monounsaturated Fat 2 g
Cholesterol 47 mg		Polyunsaturated Fat 2 g

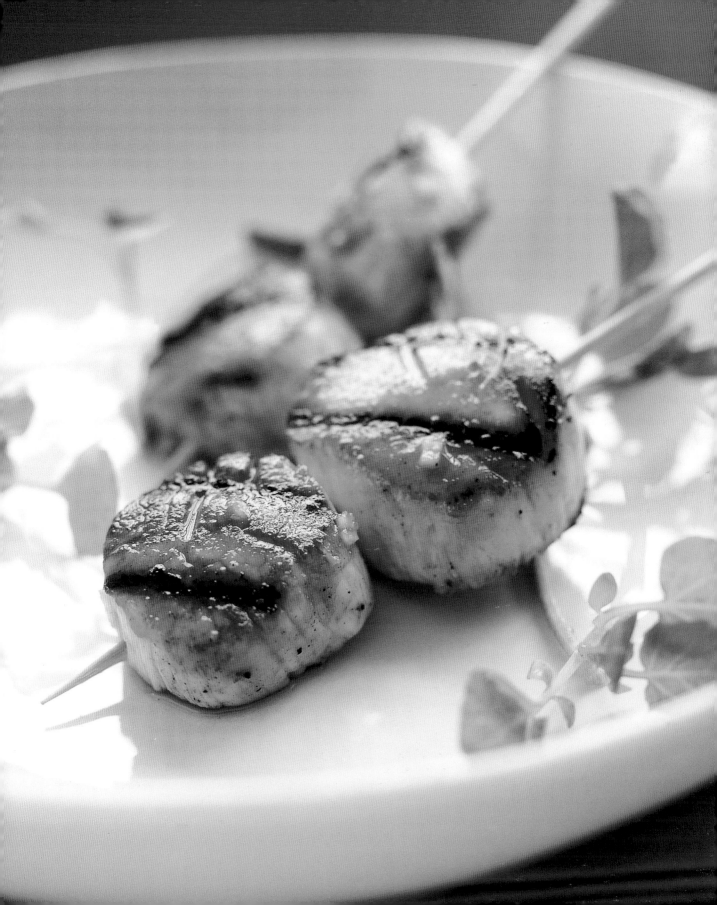

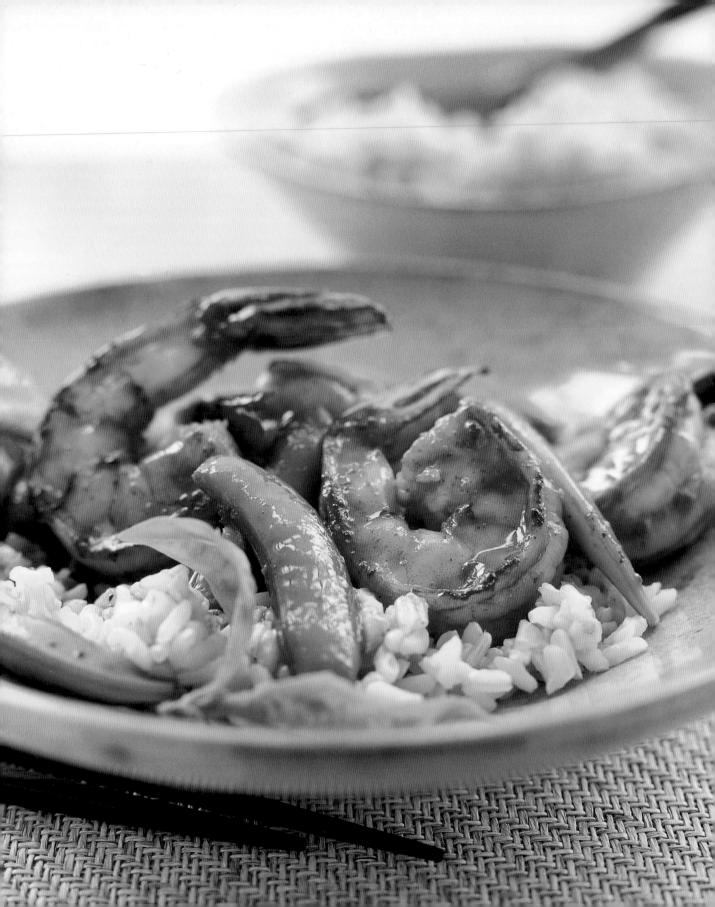

THAI PRAWNS WITH RICE

DIABETIC EXCHANGES

2 starch	0 fruit	0 milk
1½ vegetable	2½ protein	½ fat

SERVES 4

Crisp sugar snap peas and sweet fresh prawns are paired in this dish with classic Thai seasonings: garlic, chilli, basil, and lime. If you can't find prepared chilli-garlic sauce (or purée), you can substitute ½ teaspoon chilli flakes and 1 more clove of garlic, crushed.

In a saucepan, combine the rice and water. Bring to a boil over medium-high heat. Reduce the heat to low, cover, and simmer for about 45 minutes until the water is absorbed and the rice is tender. Transfer to a large bowl and keep warm.

While the rice is cooking, in a large non-stick frying pan, heat the sesame oil over medium-high heat. Add the prawns, garlic, and chilli-garlic sauce. Toss and stir for about 2 minutes until the mixture is sizzling. Add the sugar snap peas and continue to toss and stir, for 3–4 minutes, until the prawns are opaque and the peas are tender-crisp.

In a small bowl, combine the stock, soy sauce, and cornflour and stir to mix well. Add the stock mixture to the prawn mixture and toss until the sauce thickens, for about 1 minute. Divide the cooked rice among individual plates and top with the prawn mixture. Drizzle with the lime juice and garnish with the basil, if desired.

60 g (2½ oz) long-grain brown rice

375 ml (12 fl oz) water

1 teaspoon dark sesame oil

375 g (12 oz) large prawns, peeled and deveined

3 cloves garlic, crushed

2 teaspoons chilli-garlic sauce

225 g (8 oz) small sugar snap peas, trimmed

125 ml (4 fl oz) fat-free, no-salt-added chicken stock

1 tablespoon low-sodium soy sauce

2 teaspoons cornflour

2 tablespoons fresh lime juice

2 tablespoons chopped fresh basil (optional)

NUTRIENT ANALYSIS FOR ONE SERVING

Calories 295	**Carbohydrates** 40 g	**Total Fat** 4 g
Protein 24 g	**Fibre** 5 g	**Saturated Fat** 1 g
Sodium 471 mg	**Sugars** 6 g	**Monounsaturated Fat** 1 g
Cholesterol 129 mg		**Polyunsaturated Fat** 1 g

CHICKEN WITH CARAMELIZED ONIONS

SERVES 4

4 teaspoons olive oil or sunflower oil

1 large onion, thinly sliced

½ teaspoon salt

85 ml (2½ fl oz) fat-free, no-salt-added chicken stock

½ tablespoon balsamic vinegar

1 teaspoon wholegrain mustard

¼ teaspoon freshly ground black pepper

4 skinless, boneless chicken breasts, 100 g (4 oz) each

1½ tablespoons chopped fresh thyme, plus several sprigs for garnish (optional)

As onions cook slowly, their natural sharpness fades. After enough slow cooking, the onions caramelize – that is, they become dark, sweet, and rich with a texture like that of jam.

In a large non-stick frying pan, heat 3 teaspoons of the oil over medium-low heat. Add the onion and cook for about 20–30 minutes, stirring frequently, until the onion is golden brown. (Do not let the onion burn.) Stir in ¼ teaspoon of the salt.

In a small saucepan over medium-low heat, combine the stock, vinegar, and mustard and whisk to blend. Add the onion and a little pepper and cook for 4–5 minutes until the liquid is reduced by half. Remove from the heat and keep warm.

Place the chicken breasts between 2 sheets of heavy-duty cling film. With a meat mallet or rolling pin, pound the breasts to an even 6-mm (¼-in) thickness. Sprinkle the pounded chicken with the remaining salt and the pepper. Place the chopped thyme in a shallow dish. Dredge the chicken in the thyme, pressing to make the leaves stick.

In the same large non-stick pan used for the onion, heat the remaining 1 teaspoon oil over medium-high heat. Add the chicken and cook, about 2–3 minutes per side, turning once, until opaque throughout.

To serve, place the chicken on individual plates and top with the onion mixture. Garnish each with a sprig of thyme, if desired.

NUTRIENT ANALYSIS FOR ONE SERVING

Calories 191	Carbohydrates 6 g	Total Fat 6 g
Protein 27 g	Fibre 1 g	Saturated Fat 1 g
Sodium 390 mg	Sugars 4 g	Monounsaturated Fat 4 g
Cholesterol 66 mg		Polyunsaturated Fat 1 g

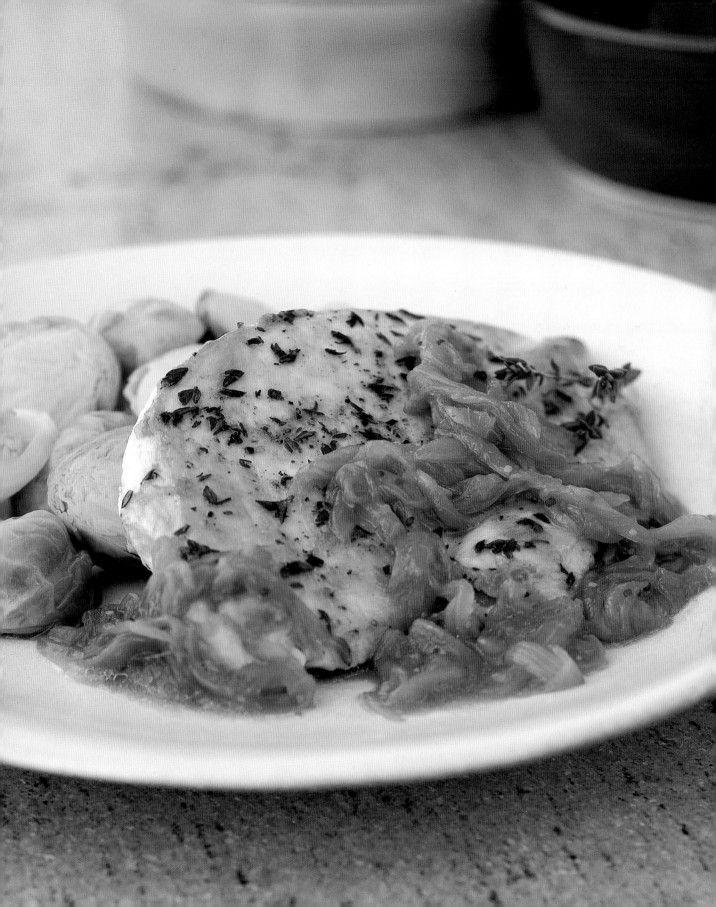

6g

CHICKEN BREASTS STUFFED WITH TOMATO & BASIL

SERVES 4

- 25 g (1 oz) fresh mozzarella cheese, chopped
- 4 large basil leaves, chopped
- 1 small plum tomato, seeded and finely chopped
- ½ teaspoon salt
- 4 skinless, boneless chicken breasts, 100 g (4 oz) each
- 3 tablespoons plain flour
- ¼ teaspoon paprika
- ¼ teaspoon freshly ground black pepper
- 1 tablespoon olive oil or sunflower oil

Simply slice pockets into chicken breasts to add a tasty stuffing. Here, the chicken breasts are filled with chopped tomatoes, mozzarella, and fresh basil. Try wholemeal bread crumbs with chopped nuts and parsley for another healthy stuffing.

In a small bowl, combine the mozzarella cheese, chopped basil, tomato, and ¼ teaspoon of the salt.

Place 1 chicken breast on a chopping board and hold it flat with your hand. Using a small, sharp knife, cut a horizontal slice in the side of the breast to make a pocket as large as you can without cutting through the other side. Repeat with the remaining chicken breasts. Spoon one-quarter of the cheese-tomato mixture into each pocket and pin the pocket closed with a cocktail stick.

In a shallow bowl, combine the flour, paprika, pepper, and the remaining ½ teaspoon of the salt. Dredge the stuffed chicken breasts in the flour mixture to coat well.

In a large frying pan, heat the oil over medium-high heat. Add the stuffed chicken breasts and cook 4–5 minutes per side, turning once, until opaque throughout and tender. Transfer to a warmed serving platter. Remove the cocktail sticks and serve immediately.

NUTRIENT ANALYSIS FOR ONE SERVING

Calories 201	Carbohydrates 6 g	Total Fat 6 g
Protein 28 g	Fibre 0 g	Saturated Fat 2 g
Sodium 396 mg	Sugars 1 g	Monounsaturated Fat 3 g
Cholesterol 71 mg		Polyunsaturated Fat 1 g

TURKEY & VEGETABLE MEATLOAF

CARB COUNT 14g

DIABETIC EXCHANGES
| ½ starch | 0 fruit | 0 milk |
| ½ vegetable | 3 protein | 0 fat |

SERVES 6

Diced and grated fresh vegetables and a sprinkling of oats help keep this meatloaf deliciously moist. Accompanied by Mashed Sweet Potatoes (page 107) and steamed green beans, it's comfort food at its best. Slice any leftovers for meatloaf sandwiches.

Preheat the oven to 180°C (350°F).

In a large bowl, combine the oats and chicken stock. Let stand for 20–25 minutes until most of the liquid is absorbed. Add the minced turkey, onion, carrot, mushrooms, tomato purée, thyme, sage, egg whites, salt, and pepper. Mix with a large spoon or by hand until well blended.

Place the turkey mixture in a non-stick 23 x 12.5-cm (9 x 5-in) loaf tin, pressing down gently to fit. Bake about 50–55 minutes until no longer pink inside and the juice runs clear when pierced with a knife. Let stand for 15 minutes before slicing.

- 100 g (4 oz) old-fashioned rolled oats
- 125 ml (4 fl oz) fat-free, no-salt-added chicken stock
- 500 g (1 lb 2 oz) lean minced turkey
- ½ onion, coarsely chopped
- ½ large carrot, coarsely grated
- 175 g (6 oz) chestnut or button mushrooms, coarsley chopped
- 4 tablespoons tomato purée
- 1 tablespoon chopped fresh thyme or 1 teaspoon dried thyme
- 1 tablespoon chopped fresh sage or 1 teaspoon dried sage
- 2 egg whites, lightly beaten
- ½ teaspoon salt
- ½ teaspoon freshly ground black pepper

NUTRIENT ANALYSIS FOR ONE SERVING

Calories 222	**Carbohydrates** 14 g	**Total Fat** 8 g
Protein 25 g	**Fibre** 3 g	**Saturated Fat** 2 g
Sodium 329 mg	**Sugars** 2 g	**Monounsaturated Fat** 5 g
Cholesterol 59 mg		**Polyunsaturated Fat** 1 g

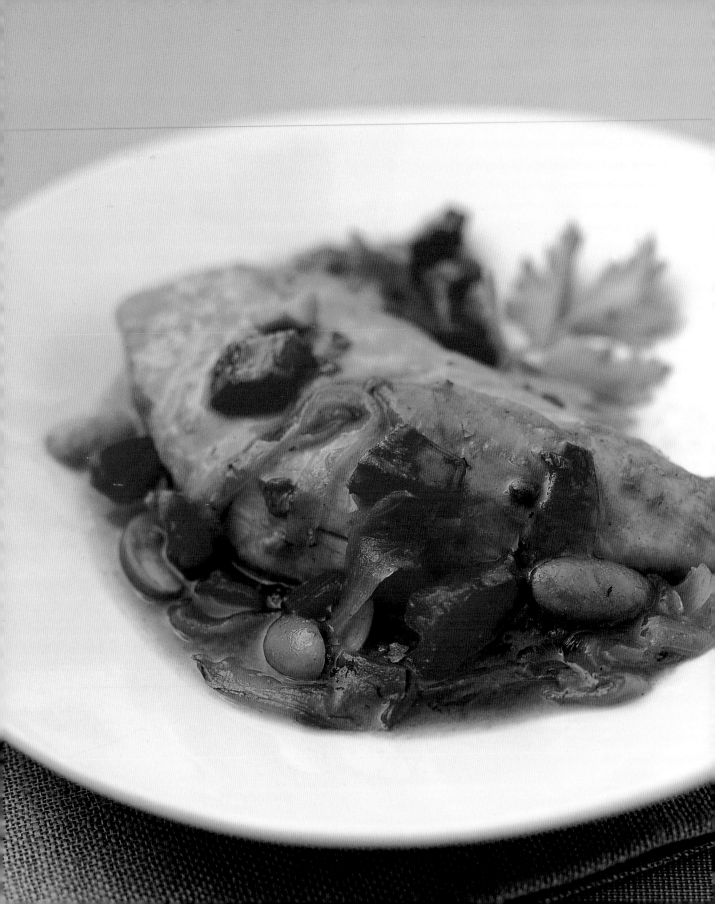

BRAISED CHICKEN WITH TOMATOES & OLIVES

SERVES 4

Green olives, capers, oregano, and other seasonings are combined with a bit of Marsala, a sweet wine from Sicily, to give this savoury chicken dish a Mediterranean character. For a complete meal, pair it with wholemeal bread and a salad.

In a shallow bowl, combine the flour, oregano, black pepper, and chilli flakes. Dredge the chicken pieces in the flour mixture.

In a large saucepan or flameproof casserole coated generously with cooking spray, heat the olive oil over medium-high heat. Add the chicken and cook for about 5 minutes until browned on all sides. Transfer the chicken to a platter. Add the onion to the pan and sauté for about 4 minutes until it begins to soften and brown. Add the tomatoes and sauté for 2 minutes. Stir in the stock and Marsala, stirring with a wooden spoon to scrape up any browned bits. Return the chicken to the pan. Bring to a boil, reduce the heat to low, cover, and simmer for 45–50 minutes, stirring occasionally, until the chicken is tender. Stir in the chopped parsley, olives, capers, and salt.

To serve, place 1 chicken breast piece and 1 chicken thigh in warmed individual bowls. Top with the sauce and garnish with a sprig of parsley, if desired.

4 tablespoons plain flour

1 teaspoon dried oregano

¼ teaspoon freshly ground black pepper

⅛ teaspoon chilli flakes

2 small bone-in chicken breast halves, about 175 g (6 oz) each, skinned and cut in half crosswise

4 bone-in chicken thighs, about 175 g (6 oz) each, skinned

Cooking spray

1½ teaspoons olive oil

1 large onion, sliced

2 small plum tomatoes, chopped

125 ml (4 fl oz) fat-free, no-salt-added chicken stock

125 ml (4 fl oz) Marsala or dry red wine

4 tablespoons chopped fresh parsley, plus sprigs for garnish (optional)

25 g (1 oz) small pitted green olives, halved

1 tablespoon capers, rinsed

⅛ teaspoon salt

NUTRIENT ANALYSIS FOR ONE SERVING

Calories 221	**Carbohydrates** 14 g	**Total Fat** 7 g
Protein 25 g	**Fibre** 2 g	**Saturated Fat** 2 g
Sodium 356 mg	**Sugars** 5 g	**Monounsaturated Fat** 3 g
Cholesterol 67 mg		**Polyunsaturated Fat** 1 g

PAN-SEARED DUCK BREAST WITH ORANGE SAUCE

2 teaspoons grated orange zest

175 ml (6 fl oz) fresh orange juice

4 skinless, boneless duck or chicken breasts, about 100 g (4 oz) each

¼ teaspoon salt, plus ⅛ teaspoon

¼ teaspoon freshly ground black pepper

1 tablespoon olive oil or sunflower oil

125 ml (4 fl oz) fat-free, no-salt-added chicken stock

1 tablespoon chopped fresh chives

1 tablespoon chopped fresh parsley

1 teaspoon chopped fresh tarragon

Skinless chicken breast is a mainstay for healthy eaters, but skinless duck breast is actually leaner – and more flavourful. Duck has also become easier to find in supermarkets. Check the weights and divide the breasts if they are too large.

In a large shallow non-metallic container or a lock-top plastic bag, combine the orange zest and 125 ml (4 fl oz) of the orange juice. Add the duck and turn to coat both sides. Cover or seal the container and refrigerate for 30 minutes, turning occasionally. Remove the duck from the marinade and pat dry with paper towels. Discard the marinade. Sprinkle the duck with ¼ teaspoon of the salt and a little pepper.

In a large non-stick frying pan, heat the oil over medium heat. Add the duck and cook about 6 minutes per side, turning once, until medium-well done, with only a hint of pink in the centre. Transfer to a platter and let stand for 5 minutes.

Add the chicken stock and the remaining orange juice to the frying pan over medium-high heat and deglaze the pan, stirring with a wooden spoon to scrape up any browned bits. Bring to a boil, reduce the heat to low, and simmer for 3–4 minutes until the mixture is reduced by one-third. Remove from the heat and stir in the chives, parsley, tarragon, the remaining salt, and the pepper.

To serve, slice each duck breast on the diagonal into thin slices. Fan the slices on a warmed serving platter and top with the sauce.

NUTRIENT ANALYSIS FOR ONE SERVING

Calories 208	Carbohydrates 4 g	Total Fat 6 g
Protein 32 g	Fibre 0 g	Saturated Fat 1 g
Sodium 353 mg	Sugars 3 g	Monounsaturated Fat 3 g
Cholesterol 162 mg		Polyunsaturated Fat 1 g

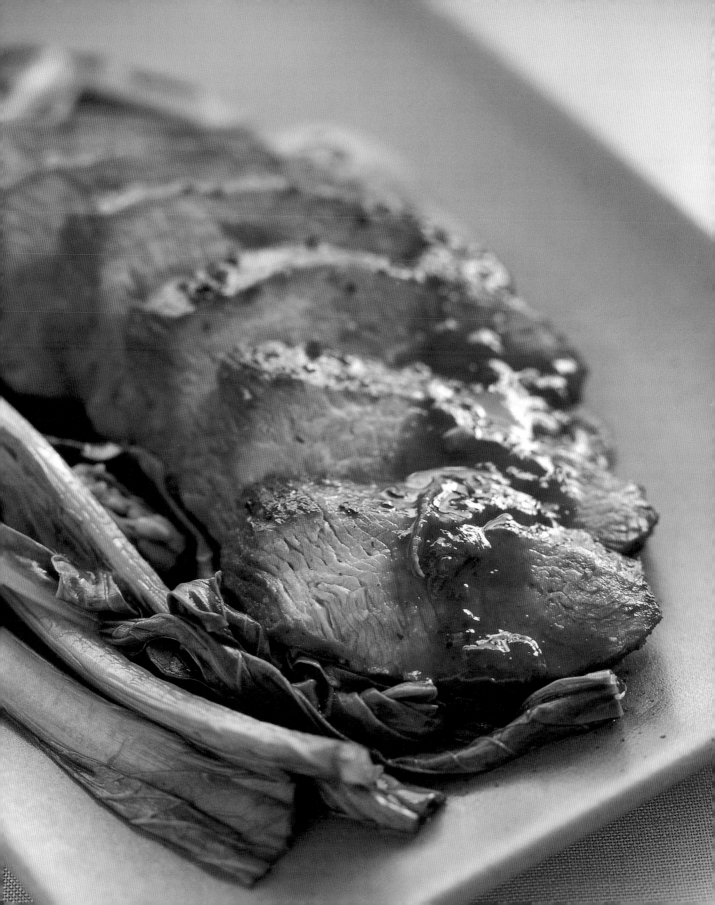

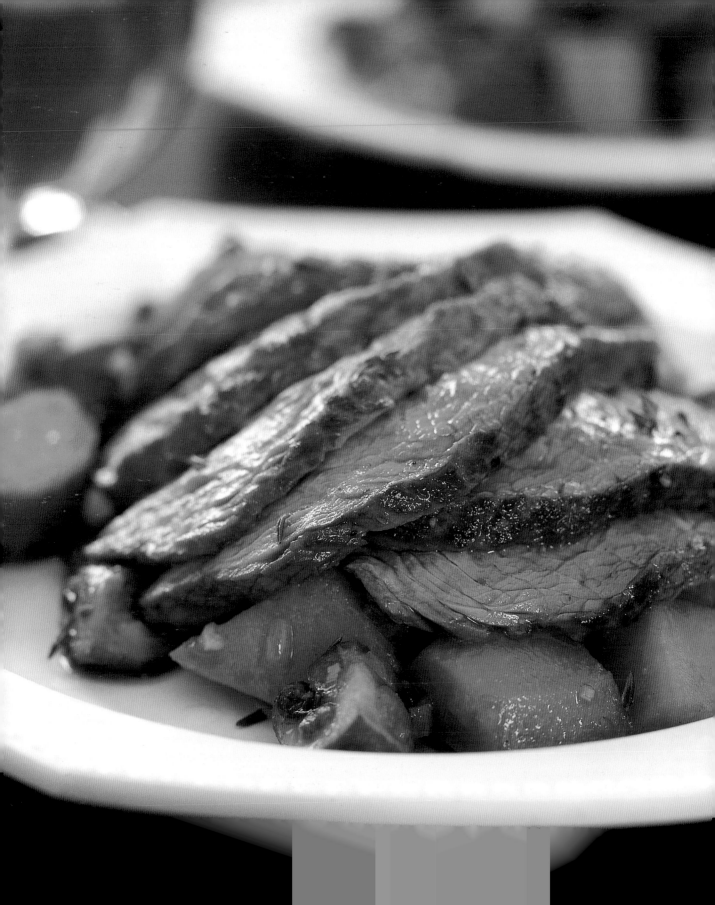

SEARED SIRLOIN WITH SWEET POTATO RAGOUT

CARB COUNT 22g

DIABETIC EXCHANGES

| 1 starch | 0 fruit | 0 milk |
| 1 vegetable | 3½ protein | 1½ fat |

SERVES 4

Rich with the flavours of garlic and thyme, this dish takes only minutes to prepare yet is elegant enough to serve to guests. Asparagus with Shallots & Blue Cheese (page 46) is an excellent complement to this hearty-but-light main course.

Combine the stock and sweet potatoes in a large deep frying pan. Bring to a simmer over medium heat, cover, and cook for 8 minutes. Add the sliced mushrooms, shallots, garlic, mustard, thyme, and a little pepper. Cook about 5 minutes, stirring frequently, until the vegetables are tender and the sauce is slightly reduced. Remove from the heat and keep warm while preparing the steak.

Heat a large non-stick frying pan over medium-high heat until hot. Place the steak in the frying pan and sprinkle with the salt and pepper. Cook for 4 minutes per side, turning once, until browned. Cut into the centre to check for doneness. Transfer the steak to a carving board.

Cut the steak across the grain into thin slices. Spoon the sweet potato ragout onto warmed individual plates; top with the sliced steak. Garnish with thyme sprigs, if desired, and serve immediately.

- 175 ml (6 fl oz) fat-free, no-salt-added beef stock
- 2 sweet potatoes, about 450 g (1 lb) total weight, cut into 1-cm (½-in) cubes
- 225 g (8 oz) chestnut or button mushrooms, brushed clean and sliced, or packaged sliced mixed fresh mushrooms, such as oyster, chestnut, and shiitake
- 2 shallots, finely chopped
- 2 cloves garlic, crushed
- 1½ tablespoons Dijon mustard
- 1½ tablespoons chopped fresh thyme, plus several thyme sprigs for garnish (optional)
- ½ teaspoon freshly ground black pepper
- 450 g (1 lb) sirloin steak, 2.5 cm (1 in) thick and trimmed of visible fat
- ¼ teaspoon salt

NUTRIENT ANALYSIS FOR ONE SERVING

Calories 289	**Carbohydrates** 22 g	**Total Fat** 9 g
Protein 30 g	**Fibre** 4 g	**Saturated Fat** 3 g
Sodium 385 mg	**Sugars** 7 g	**Monounsaturated Fat** 4 g
Cholesterol 74 mg		**Polyunsaturated Fat** 1 g

PORK LOIN WITH APPLES

DIABETIC EXCHANGES

0 starch	1 fruit	0 milk
1 vegetable	3½ protein	1½ fat

SERVES 4

1½ teaspoons paprika

1½ teaspoons dried sage or thyme

½ teaspoon salt

¼ teaspoon freshly ground black pepper

½ teaspoon ground allspice

4 boneless centre-cut pork loin chops, each about 100 g (4 oz) and 1 cm (½ in) thick, trimmed of visible fat

3 Granny Smith apples, peeled, cored, and cut into thin slices

4 shallots, chopped

125 ml (4 fl oz) unsweetened apple juice

2 teaspoons cider vinegar

1 tablespoon chopped fresh sage or thyme (optional)

Surprisingly lean, these pork loin chops can easily claim a spot on a heart-healthy menu. Granny Smith apples make an ideal partner for the pork, but you can use Fuji, Gala, or small cooking apples. Serve with steamed green beans or broccoli.

Preheat a grill to medium-high or prepare a barbecue. Position the cooking rack 10–15 cm (4–6 in) from the heat source.

In a small bowl, combine the paprika, dried sage, salt, pepper, and half of the allspice. Sprinkle the mixture over both sides of the pork chops. Cook for about 5 minutes per side, turning once, until the pork is browned on both sides and is no longer pink on the inside.

Meanwhile, in a large non-stick frying pan over high heat, combine the apples, shallots, apple juice, vinegar, and the remaining allspice. Bring to a boil, reduce the heat to medium, and cook for 10–12 minutes, stirring occasionally, until the apples are tender and the sauce is slightly reduced. Transfer the pork chops to individual plates, top with the sauce, and garnish with the fresh sage, if desired.

NUTRIENT ANALYSIS FOR ONE SERVING

Calories 268	**Carbohydrates** 24 g	**Total Fat** 9 g
Protein 25 g	**Fibre** 2 g	**Saturated Fat** 3 g
Sodium 344 mg	**Sugars** 15 g	**Monounsaturated Fat** 4 g
Cholesterol 62 mg		**Polyunsaturated Fat** 1 g

VEAL PICCATA

SERVES 4

CARB COUNT

4g

DIABETIC EXCHANGES

0 starch	0 fruit	0 milk
0 vegetable	3½ protein	½ fat

Often overlooked, veal is among the leanest meats. It is easy to cook, especially when purchased in thin cutlets. The Italian specialty called *piccata* features capers, garlic, lemon zest, and parsley. Serve it with Polenta with Garlic & Basil (page 104).

Combine the flour, salt, and pepper in a plastic or paper bag. Add the veal escalopes to the bag one at a time, shaking to coat.

In a large non-stick frying pan, heat 1 teaspoon of the olive oil over medium-high heat. Add half of the veal escalopes and cook about 2 minutes per side, turning once, until lightly browned on both sides. Transfer to a plate and set aside. Keep warm. Repeat with the remaining olive oil and the remaining veal cutlets.

In the same frying pan over medium heat, add half of the garlic and cook until fragrant, about 30 seconds. Add the stock and lemon juice and simmer for 3–4 minutes, stirring once, until the sauce is slightly reduced.

In a small bowl, combine the parsley, capers, lemon zest, and the remaining garlic. Stir the parsley mixture into the sauce. Return the veal to the frying pan and warm, turning once, just until heated through.

2 tablespoons plain flour

½ teaspoon salt

¼ teaspoon freshly ground black pepper

450 g (1 lb) veal escalopes

2 teaspoons olive oil

2 cloves garlic, crushed

125 ml (4 fl oz) fat-free, no-salt-added chicken stock

1 tablespoon fresh lemon juice

3 tablespoons chopped fresh parsley

1 tablespoon capers, rinsed

½ teaspoon grated lemon zest

NUTRIENT ANALYSIS FOR ONE SERVING

Calories 163	**Carbohydrates** 4 g	**Total Fat** 4 g
Protein 26 g	**Fibre** 0 g	**Saturated Fat** 1 g
Sodium 305 mg	**Sugars** 0 g	**Monounsaturated Fat** 2 g
Cholesterol 88 mg		**Polyunsaturated Fat** 0 g

SZECHUAN PORK STIR-FRY

DIABETIC EXCHANGES

1 starch	0 fruit	0 milk
1 vegetable	3 protein	½ fat

SERVES 4

1 pork tenderloin, about 450 g (1 lb), trimmed of visible fat

1 teaspoon crushed Szechuan peppercorns or chilli flakes

3 cloves garlic, crushed

2 teaspoons peeled and grated fresh ginger or 1 teaspoon ground ginger

1 teaspoon sunflower oil

1 red sweet pepper, cut into short, thin strips

200 g (7 oz) mangetout, halved diagonally

6 spring onions, sliced diagonally

4 tablespoons hoisin sauce

2 teaspoons toasted sesame seeds

Pork tenderloin is almost as lean as skinless chicken breast. Stir-fried with spices and vegetables, it makes a complete healthy meal with unmistakable Asian flair. Take care not to overcook the pork so it stays tender and juicy.

Slice the pork crosswise into 6-mm (¼-in) slices. Cut each slice in half. In a bowl, combine the pork, crushed peppercorns, garlic, and ginger and toss to coat; set aside.

Heat the sunflower oil in a large non-stick frying pan over medium-high heat until hot. Add the sweet pepper and cook about 2 minutes, tossing continuously, until the pepper strips start to brown. Add the mangetout and cook about 1 minute, tossing continuously, until slightly softened. Add the pork mixture and cook about 2 minutes, tossing continuously, until the mixture begins to thicken. Add the spring onions and hoisin sauce and cook 2–3 minutes, tossing continuously, until the pork is no longer pink in the centre. Transfer to a serving dish and garnish with the sesame seeds. Serve immediately.

NUTRIENT ANALYSIS FOR ONE SERVING

Calories 278	**Carbohydrates** 20 g	**Total Fat** 9 g
Protein 28 g	**Fibre** 4 g	**Saturated Fat** 3 g
Sodium 388 mg	**Sugars** 5 g	**Monounsaturated Fat** 4 g
Cholesterol 78 mg		**Polyunsaturated Fat** 2 g

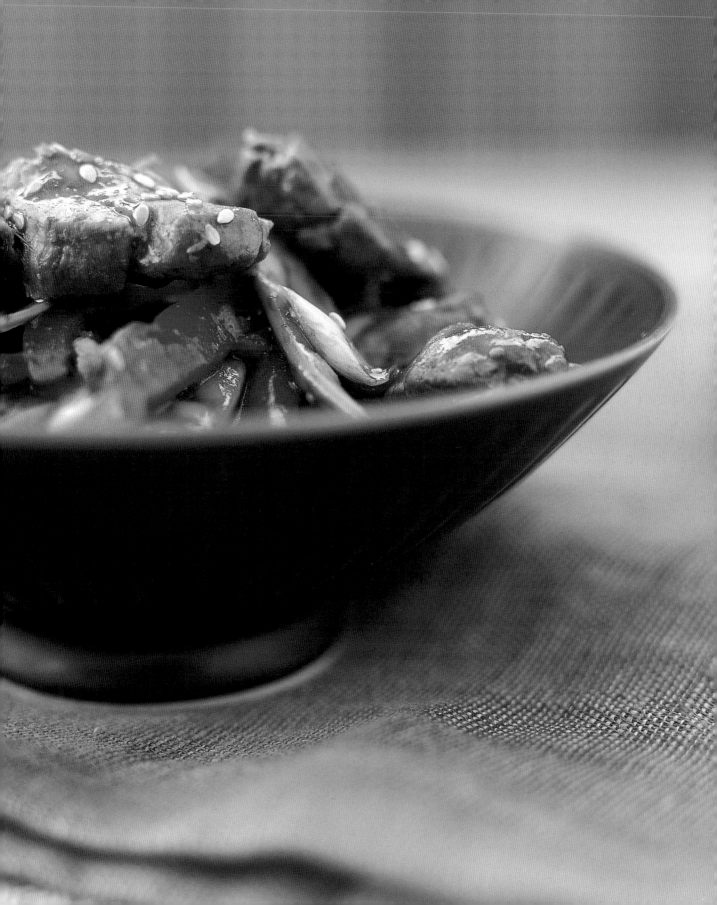

DIABETIC EXCHANGES

½ starch	0 fruit	0 milk
1½ vegetable	1 protein	1 fat

LEEK & SWEET PEPPER FRITTATA

SERVES 4

1½ teaspoons olive oil or sunflower oil

1 large leek, thinly sliced

1 small potato, peeled and grated

½ red sweet pepper, chopped

¼ teaspoon salt

2 whole eggs plus 3 egg whites

4 tablespoons skimmed milk

4 large basil leaves, chopped

¼ teaspoon freshly ground black pepper

⅛ teaspoon freshly grated nutmeg

5 g (½ oz) grated Parmesan cheese

Lightened with egg whites and skimmed milk, this easy low-fat baked omelette, or frittata, is enjoyable at any meal. You can replace the leek and red pepper with other vegetables, or add chopped smoked turkey or other cooked lean meat.

In a large non-stick frying pan with an ovenproof handle, heat the oil over medium heat. Add the sliced leek and grated potato and sauté for 8–10 minutes, until tender. Stir in the chopped sweet pepper and ⅛ teaspoon of the salt and cook for 2 minutes. Spread the vegetables evenly in the pan.

Preheat the grill.

In a bowl, whisk together the whole eggs and egg whites. Stir in the milk, basil, the remaining salt, pepper, and nutmeg. Pour the egg mixture into the pan with the vegetables and sprinkle the cheese evenly over the top. Cook about 2 minutes until slightly set.

Carefully place the pan under the grill and cook about 3 minutes until the frittata is brown and puffy and completely set. Gently slide the frittata onto a warmed serving platter and cut into wedges. Serve immediately.

NUTRIENT ANALYSIS FOR ONE SERVING

Calories 137	Carbohydrates 17 g	Total Fat 5 g
Protein 8 g	Fibre 2 g	Saturated Fat 1 g
Sodium 239 mg	Sugars 4 g	Monounsaturated Fat 2 g
Cholesterol 107 mg		Polyunsaturated Fat 1 g

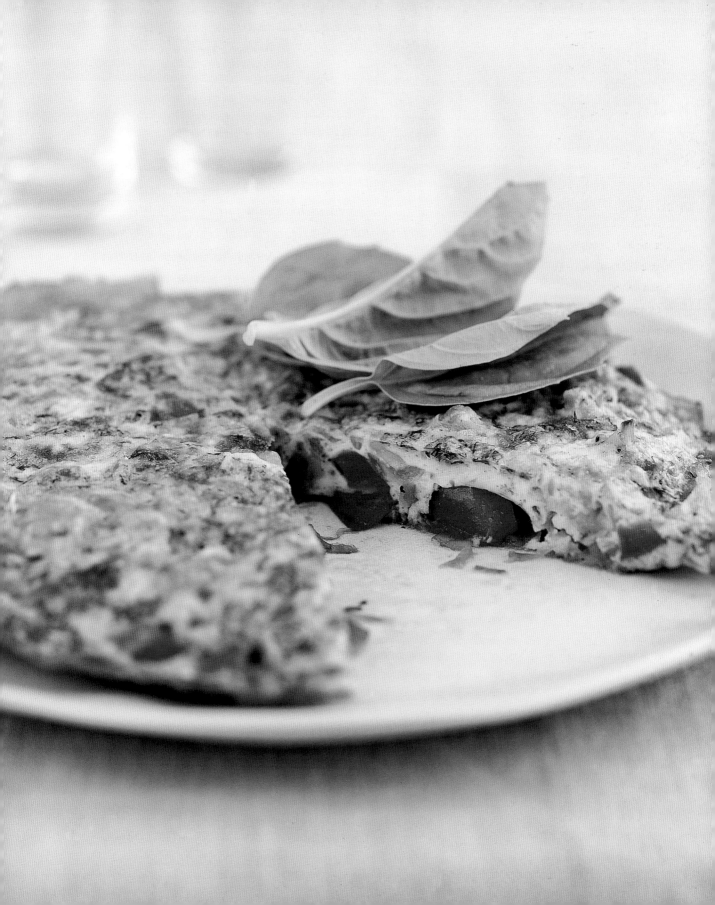

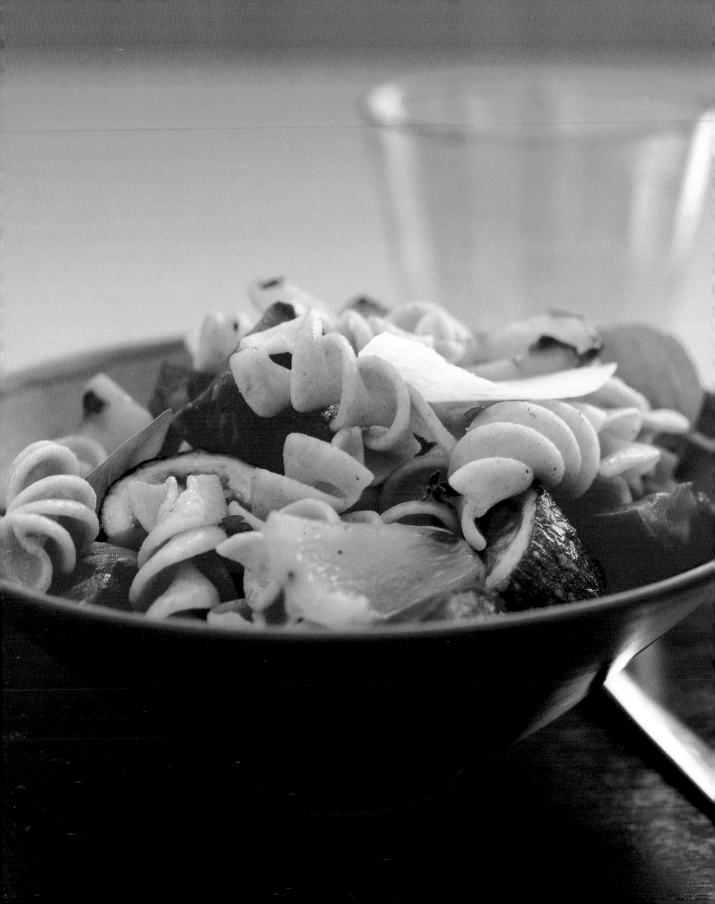

PASTA WITH ROASTED VEGETABLES

CARB COUNT 58g

DIABETIC EXCHANGES
3 starch	0 fruit	0 milk
2 vegetable	2 protein	2 fat

SERVES 4

Roasting vegetables gives them a smoky sweetness that's irresistible with pasta. To make the most nutritious version of this dish, use 100-per cent wholewheat pasta. But if you want a milder flavour, look for 50-per cent wholewheat pasta.

Preheat the oven to 200°C (400°F).

Arrange the chunks of courgette, pepper, and onion on a non-stick baking sheet. Drizzle the sheet with 2 tablespoons of the olive oil. Sprinkle with ¼ teaspoon of the salt and a little pepper. Toss gently to mix. Add the unpeeled garlic cloves to the baking sheet and roast 20–25 minutes, until the vegetables are nearly tender and beginning to brown. Add the tomatoes and continue to roast for 10 minutes longer.

While the tomatoes are roasting, bring a large pot three-quarters full of water to a boil. Add the pasta and cook for 10–12 minutes until *al dente*, or according to package directions. Drain the pasta thoroughly, transfer to a large bowl, and toss with the remaining olive oil.

Peel the roasted garlic and mash with a fork. Stir the garlic into the pasta. Stir the remaining roasted vegetables into the pasta. Add the parsley, chopped basil, thyme, the remaining salt, and a little pepper. Toss gently to mix.

To serve, divide the pasta mixture evenly among shallow, warmed bowls. Using a vegetable peeler, cut a curl or two of Parmesan cheese to top each serving. Garnish with a leaf of basil, if desired.

2 small courgettes, about 225 g (8 oz) total weight, cut into 2.5-cm (1-in) chunks

2 yellow sweet peppers, seeded and cut into 2.5-cm (1-in) chunks

½ onion, cut into 2.5-cm (1-in) chunks

3 tablespoons olive oil

½ teaspoon salt

¼ teaspoon freshly ground black pepper

10 cloves garlic, unpeeled

8 plum tomatoes, about 450 g (1 lb) total weight, seeded and coarsely chopped

225 g (8 oz) wholewheat or 50-per cent wholewheat pasta spirals or other dry pasta

3 tablespoons chopped fresh parsley

3 tablespoons chopped fresh basil, plus 4 leaves for garnish (optional)

½ tablespoon chopped fresh thyme

25-g (1-oz) chunk Parmesan cheese

NUTRIENT ANALYSIS FOR ONE SERVING

Calories 380	**Carbohydrates** 58 g	**Total Fat** 13 g
Protein 14 g	**Fibre** 5 g	**Saturated Fat** 3 g
Sodium 409 mg	**Sugars** 9 g	**Monounsaturated Fat** 8 g
Cholesterol 4 mg		**Polyunsaturated Fat** 2 g

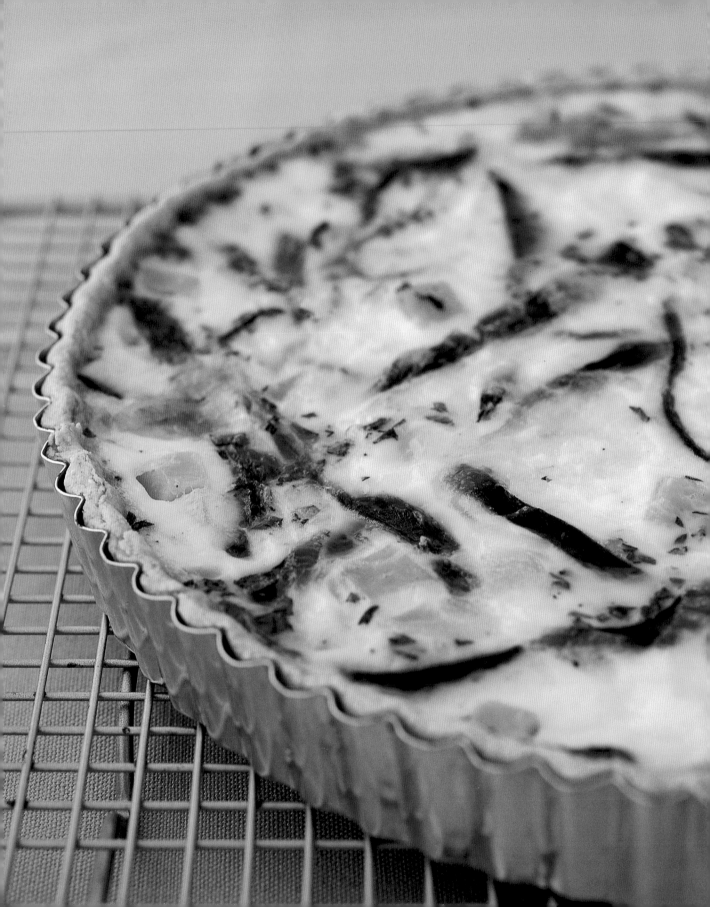

WINTER SQUASH TART

CARB COUNT **35**g

DIABETIC EXCHANGES
| 1½ starch | 0 fruit | 0 milk |
| 1 vegetable | 1 protein | 1½ fat |

SERVES 4

Chillies add a touch of spiciness to this healthy tart. Use red or yellow sweet peppers in place of the green pepper, if you like, and add a pinch of cayenne pepper.

Preheat the grill. Flatten the pepper halves with your hand. Grill the pepper for 5–6 minutes until the skin blackens. Place the pepper in a small bowl, cover with cling film, and let stand about 15 minutes until the skin loosens. Peel and discard the skin. Slice the pepper into thin strips.

In a large bowl, combine the wholemeal and plain flours, polenta, baking powder, and ⅛ teaspoon of the salt. Add 4 tablespoons of the water and the oil to the flour mixture and stir until blended. Turn the dough out onto a floured surface and knead 4 or 5 times. Press the dough into a 10-cm (4-in) round, place between sheets of cling film, and refrigerate for 15 minutes. Roll the dough, still covered, into a 25-cm (10-in) round. Transfer the round to the freezer and chill for 5 minutes or until the cling film can be easily removed.

Preheat the oven to 190°C (375°F). Press the rolled crust into a 23-cm (9-in) quiche pan coated with cooking spray, pinching the edges to fit. Bake the crust about 8 minutes until brown. Cool on a wire rack.

Place the squash and chopped chilli in a microwave steamer with the remaining water. Cover and microwave on high 4–5 minutes until tender. Drain. Spoon the squash into the crust and spread evenly. Arrange the sweet pepper strips on top. In a bowl, whisk together the egg, egg whites, milk, oregano, the remaining salt, and pepper. Pour the egg mixture over the vegetables in the crust. Sprinkle with the cheese. Bake 20–25 minutes until fully set.

1 green sweet pepper, halved and seeded

60 g (2½ oz) wholemeal flour

40 g (1½ oz) plain flour

4 tablespoons stone-ground polenta

1 teaspoon baking powder

⅛ teaspoon salt, plus ¼ teaspoon

125 ml (4 fl oz) water

1½ tablespoons olive oil or sunflower oil

Cooking spray

225 g (8 oz) butternut or acorn squash, peeled and chopped

1 red chilli, seeded and chopped

1 whole egg plus 2 egg whites

125 ml (4 fl oz) skimmed milk

2 tablespoons chopped fresh oregano or ¾ teaspoon dried oregano

¼ teaspoon freshly ground black pepper

25 g (1 oz) Cheddar cheese, grated

NUTRIENT ANALYSIS FOR ONE SERVING

Calories 244	**Carbohydrates** 35 g	**Total Fat** 8 g
Protein 10 g	**Fibre** 5 g	**Saturated Fat** 2 g
Sodium 499 mg	**Sugars** 4 g	**Monounsaturated Fat** 5 g
Cholesterol 79 mg		**Polyunsaturated Fat** 1 g

39g

SPINACH & GARLIC LASAGNE

SERVES 6

1 tablespoon olive oil or sunflower oil

15 cloves garlic, thinly sliced

175 g (6 oz) baby spinach leaves

¼ teaspoon salt

2 eggs, lightly beaten

225 g (8 oz) low-fat cottage cheese

225 g (8 oz) low-fat ricotta cheese

3 tablespoons finely chopped toasted walnuts (page 138)

3 tablespoons chopped fresh parsley

3 tablespoons chopped fresh chives

4 tablespoons chopped fresh basil

500 ml (18 fl oz) skimmed milk

40 g (1½ oz) plain flour

¼ teaspoon freshly ground black pepper

Cooking spray

9 pre-cooked sheets wholemeal lasagne

1 large plum tomato, thinly sliced

15 g (½ oz) grated Parmesan cheese

Preheat the oven to 190°C (375°F). In a large frying pan, heat ½ tablespoon of the oil over medium heat. Add the garlic and sauté 1–2 minutes, until lightly browned. Transfer the garlic to a small plate. Add half of the spinach to the pan. Sauté 2–3 minutes until the spinach wilts. Stir in ⅛ teaspoon of the salt and transfer the cooked spinach to a large bowl. Add the remaining oil and spinach to the pan. Repeat, sautéing until the spinach wilts. Stir in the remaining salt; transfer the spinach to the same bowl. When the spinach has cooled, add the eggs, cottage cheese, half of the sautéed garlic, the ricotta, toasted walnuts, parsley, chives, and 1 tablespoon of the basil. Toss gently to mix well. Set aside.

In a saucepan over medium heat, combine the milk, flour, and remaining garlic and whisk until blended. Cook 8–10 minutes, stirring constantly, until thickened. Remove from heat and stir in the remaining 3 tablespoons basil and the pepper.

Lightly coat a 23 x 33-cm (9 x 13-in) baking dish with cooking spray. Spread a quarter of the garlic sauce in the dish. Arrange 3 lasagne sheets lengthwise over the sauce and spread half of the spinach-cheese mixture on top. Top with another quarter of the sauce. Repeat with the remaining lasagne sheets, the remaining spinach-cheese mixture, and another quarter of the sauce, beginning and ending with lasagne sheets. Spread the remaining sauce over the lasagne sheets. Arrange the tomato slices on the coated lasagne sheets and sprinkle with the Parmesan.

Cover with aluminium foil and bake for 15 minutes. Uncover and continue to bake about 20 minutes longer until the noodles are tender and the sauce is bubbly. Let stand for 15 minutes before serving.

NUTRIENT ANALYSIS FOR ONE SERVING

Calories 350	Carbohydrates 39 g	Total Fat 12 g
Protein 24 g	Fibre 5 g	Saturated Fat 4 g
Sodium 493 mg	Sugars 8 g	Monounsaturated Fat 4 g
Cholesterol 90 mg		Polyunsaturated Fat 3 g

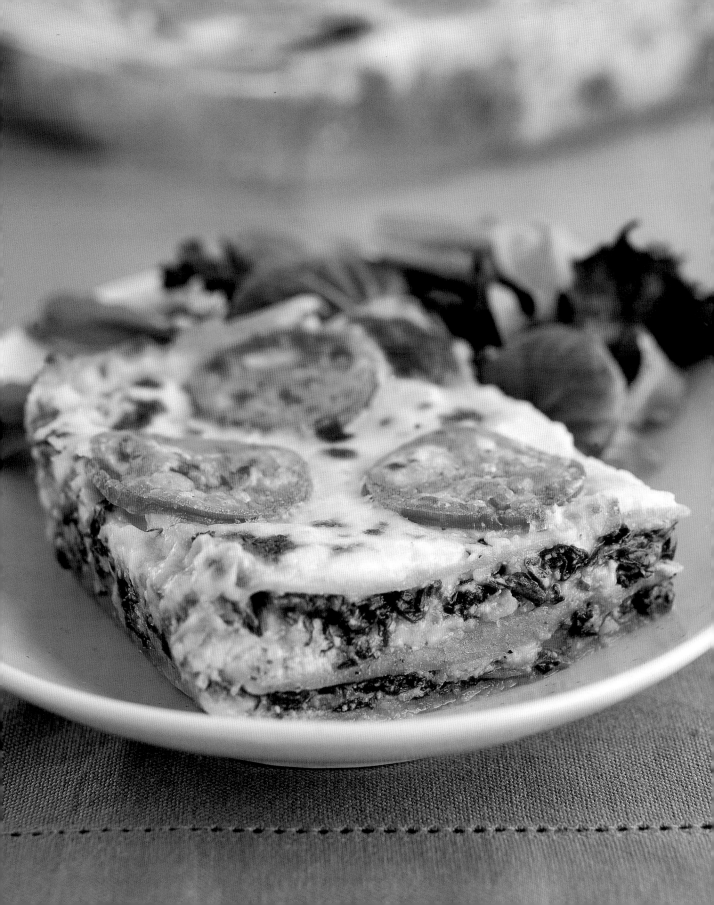

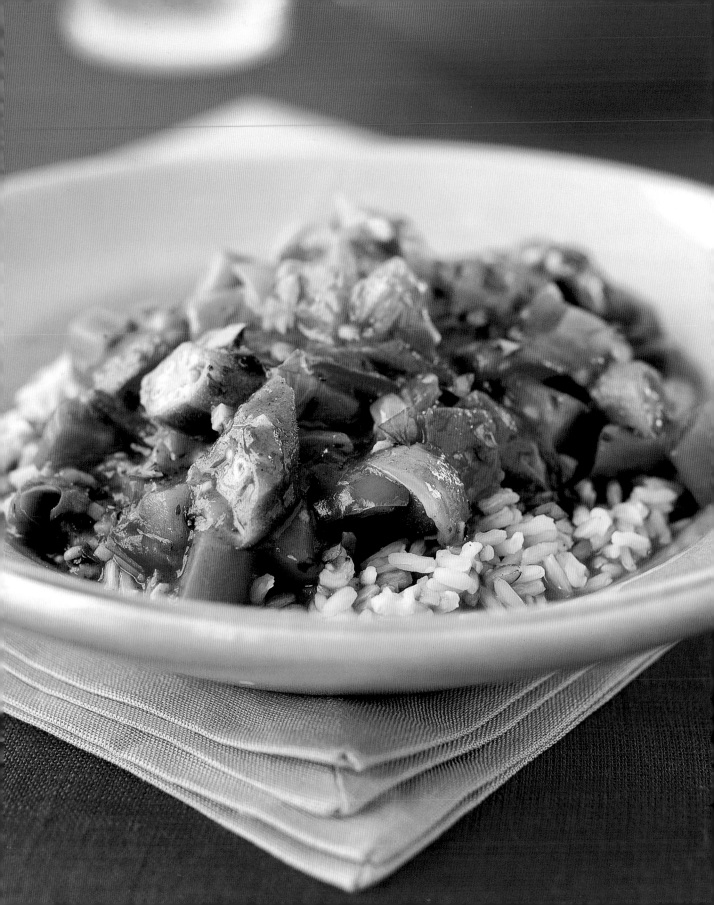

VEGETABLE GUMBO

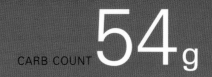

SERVES 4

DIABETIC EXCHANGES

2½ starch	0 fruit	0 milk
3 vegetable	1½ protein	1 fat

Sprinklings of three kinds of pepper give this contemporary New Orleans gumbo an alluring spiciness. Filé powder – a mild seasoning made of sassafras leaves – is a traditional thickener for gumbos and other stews, but you can leave it out.

In a saucepan, combine the rice, water, and ¼ teaspoon of the salt. Bring to a boil. Reduce the heat to low, cover, and simmer about 45 minutes until the water is absorbed and the rice is tender. Transfer to a large bowl and keep warm.

While the rice is cooking, in a large heavy saucepan, heat the sunflower oil over medium heat. Add the flour and cook about 7 minutes, stirring often, until the flour is golden brown. Add the sweet pepper, onion, carrots, and garlic and stir to mix well. Cover, raise the heat to high, and cook for 3 minutes. Uncover and stir in the stock, thyme, paprika, white pepper, black pepper, cayenne, and the remaining salt. Cover and bring to a boil over high heat. Reduce the heat to medium-low and simmer, covered, about 15 minutes, until the vegetables are tender. Stir in the okra and continue to simmer, covered, 5 minutes longer. Stir in the filé powder, if desired.

Divide the rice among individual bowls. Top each serving with the gumbo and sprinkle with the parsley.

- 175 g (6 oz) brown rice
- 500 ml (18 fl oz) water
- ½ teaspoon salt
- 1 tablespoon sunflower oil
- 2 tablespoons plain flour
- 1 large green or red sweet pepper, coarsely chopped
- 1 onion, coarsely chopped
- 275 g (10 oz) carrots, chopped or sliced
- 4 cloves garlic, crushed
- 750 ml (1¼ pt) fat-free, no-salt-added chicken or vegetable stock
- 1 tablespoon chopped fresh thyme or 1 teaspoon dried thyme
- 1 teaspoon paprika
- ¼ teaspoon ground white pepper
- ¼ teaspoon freshly ground black pepper
- ⅛ teaspoon cayenne pepper
- 1 package frozen pre-cut okra, thawed, about 225 g (8 oz)
- 1 teaspoon filé powder (optional)
- 4 tablespoons chopped fresh parsley

NUTRIENT ANALYSIS FOR ONE SERVING

Calories 307	**Carbohydrates** 54 g	**Total Fat** 5 g
Protein 11 g	**Fibre** 7 g	**Saturated Fat** 1 g
Sodium 459 mg	**Sugars** 8 g	**Monounsaturated Fat** 3 g
Cholesterol 0 mg		**Polyunsaturated Fat** 2 g

BEAN TOSTADAS WITH SWEET ONIONS

2 teaspoons sunflower oil

1 large Spanish onion, thinly sliced and separated into rings

4 corn tortillas, 15–18 cm (6–7 in) in diameter

One 400-g (15-oz) tin no-salt-added haricot, borlotti, or red kidney beans, rinsed and drained

125 ml (4 fl oz) fat-free, no-salt-added vegetable or chicken stock

4 plum tomatoes, chopped

2 green chillies, seeded and chopped

3 cloves garlic, thinly sliced

1 teaspoon ground cumin

½ teaspoon salt

50 g (2 oz) Cheshire or feta cheese, crumbled

4 tablespoons chopped fresh coriander

Naturally high in protein and in heart-healthy fibre and folate, beans form the centrepiece of this nutrient-rich and tasty dish. Black beans are the traditional beans in this dish, but other beans can be used. You can substitute 100 g (4 oz) dried black beans for the tinned beans. (For tips on cooking dried beans, see page 135.)

Preheat the oven to 200°C (400°F).

In a large non-stick frying pan, heat 1 teaspoon of the sunflower oil over medium-high heat and add the onion rings. Cover and cook about 4 minutes until golden brown. Uncover and stir well. Reduce the heat to medium and continue cooking 6–8 minutes longer until the onion is soft and deep golden brown. Set aside and keep warm.

Place the tortillas on a baking sheet and brush them with the remaining 1 teaspoon oil. Bake for 5 minutes. Turn the tortillas over and continue baking 7–8 minutes until crisp. Remove from the heat and set aside.

Meanwhile, in a saucepan over medium heat, combine the beans, stock, tomatoes, chillies, garlic, cumin, and salt. Simmer for about 10 minutes, uncovered, until most of the liquid is absorbed. Place the baked tortillas on individual plates and top with the bean mixture, sautéed onion, cheese, and coriander, dividing evenly. Serve immediately.

NUTRIENT ANALYSIS FOR ONE SERVING

Calories 278	**Carbohydrates** 41 g	**Total Fat** 8 g
Protein 13 g	**Fibre** 8 g	**Saturated Fat** 3 g
Sodium 499 mg	**Sugars** 9 g	**Monounsaturated Fat** 3 g
Cholesterol 13 mg		**Polyunsaturated Fat** 1 g

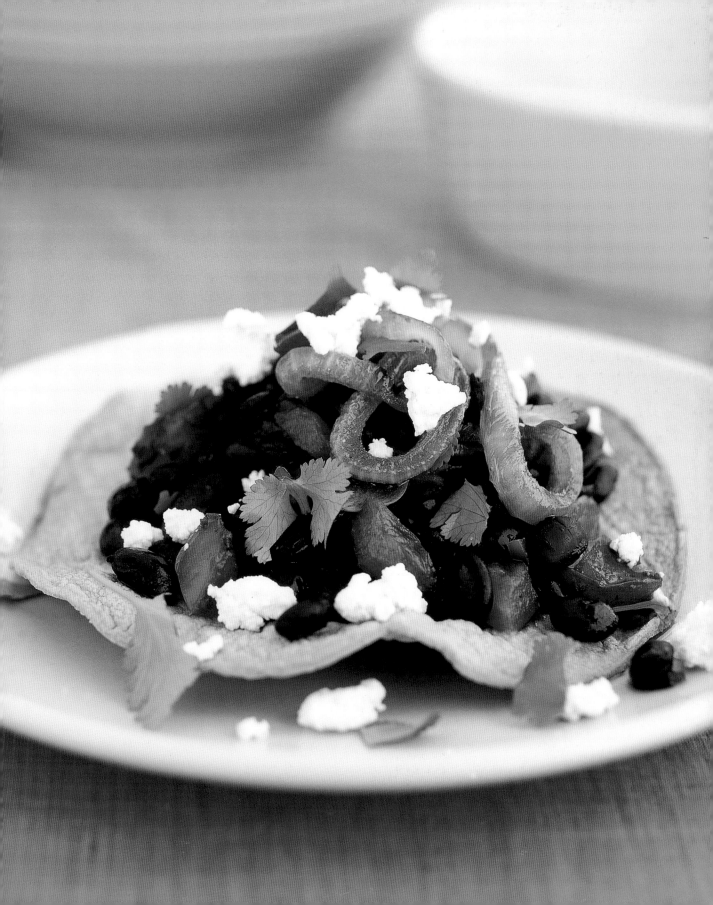

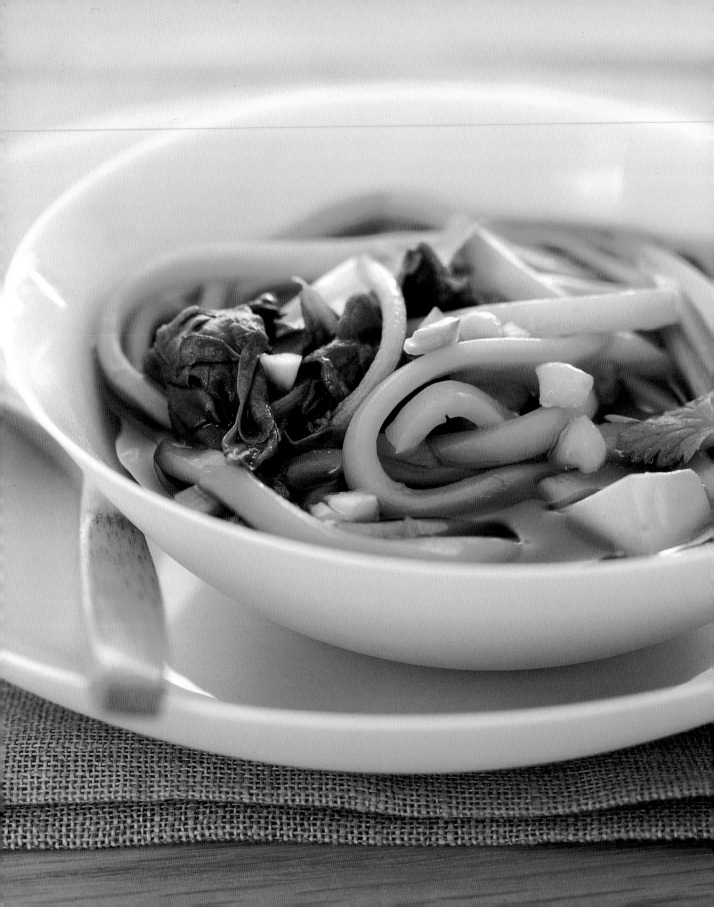

CHINESE NOODLES WITH SPINACH & TOFU

CARB COUNT **55**g

DIABETIC EXCHANGES

2½ starch   0 fruit   ½ other carbs
1 vegetable 2½ protein 1½ fat

SERVES 4

If you like Asian food, you will appreciate the complex mix of flavours in this soup. Preparing the ingredients takes a little time, but the soup comes together quickly. Look for the noodles and sesame oil in the Asian food section of your supermarket.

In a saucepan, bring the water to a boil, add the noodles, and return to the boil. Boil for 4 minutes until the noodles are tender but still slightly firm. Drain thoroughly.

While the noodles are cooking, heat the sesame oil in a wok or large frying pan over medium heat. Add the garlic and ginger and sauté about 1 minute until fragrant. Add the stock, carrot, and teriyaki sauce and bring to a simmer. Reduce the heat to low and simmer about 2 minutes until the carrot is tender. Stir in the spinach and cook for about 1 minute until wilted. Stir in the tofu and heat through. Add the cooked noodles and toss well to mix. Transfer the soup to shallow serving bowls and top with the coriander and chopped peanuts.

500 ml (18 fl oz) water

225 g (8 oz) Chinese egg noodles

2 teaspoons dark sesame oil

4 cloves garlic, crushed

2 teaspoons fresh ginger, peeled and grated

500 ml (18 fl oz) fat-free, no-salt-added chicken or vegetable stock

1 carrot, thinly sliced or cut into matchsticks

85 ml (2½ fl oz) low-sodium teriyaki sauce

75 g (3 oz) packed baby spinach or torn spinach leaves

275–325 g (10–11 oz) extra-firm tofu, drained, cut into 2.5-cm (1-in) cubes

4 tablespoons chopped fresh coriander

3 tablespoons chopped unsalted dry-roasted peanuts

NUTRIENT ANALYSIS FOR ONE SERVING

Calories 369	**Carbohydrates** 55 g	**Total Fat** 8 g
Protein 19 g	**Fibre** 3 g	**Saturated Fat** 1 g
Sodium 600 mg	**Sugars** 7 g	**Monounsaturated Fat** 3 g
Cholesterol 0 mg		**Polyunsaturated Fat** 3 g

SPICY RICE & VEGETABLES WITH FRESH CORIANDER

DIABETIC EXCHANGES

4 starch	0 fruit	0 milk
1 vegetable	1 protein	2½ fat

SERVES 4

- 250 g (9 oz) long-grain brown rice
- 750 ml (1¼ pt) water
- 1 bay leaf
- ¼ teaspoon salt, plus ½ teaspoon
- 150 g (5 oz) frozen garden peas, thawed
- 1 large carrot, grated
- ½ red sweet pepper, chopped
- 3 tablespoons chopped almonds
- 1½ tablespoons olive oil or sunflower oil
- 1½ teaspoons mustard seeds
- 1 teaspoon ground turmeric
- ½ teaspoon ground coriander
- ¼ teaspoon ground cinnamon
- ¼ teaspoon chilli flakes
- 4 tablespoons chopped fresh coriander, plus sprigs for garnish (optional)

Simple to prepare, this dish proves that meatless dinners can be delicious. It is based on the abundantly spiced vegetarian dishes popular in southern India. If you don't have ground turmeric on hand, simply omit it. The dish will still be rich and flavourful.

In a saucepan, combine the rice, water, bay leaf, and ¼ teaspoon of the salt. Bring to a boil over medium-high heat. Reduce the heat to low, cover tightly, and simmer for 30–35 minutes. Stir in the peas, carrot, and pepper. Cover again and continue cooking 8–10 minutes longer until the vegetables and rice are tender. Discard the bay leaf.

While the rice mixture is cooking, put the almonds in a small, dry non-stick frying pan over medium-high heat. Cook for 3–5 minutes, stirring often, until lightly toasted. Set aside.

In a large frying pan, heat the oil over medium heat. Add the mustard seeds, the remaining salt, turmeric, ground coriander, cinnamon, and chilli flakes. Sauté for 2 minutes. Stir in the rice mixture and cook for 2–3 minutes, until the mixture is heated through. Remove from the heat and stir in the chopped coriander.

To serve, divide the rice mixture among individual bowls. Sprinkle with the toasted almonds and garnish with sprigs of coriander, if desired. Serve immediately.

NUTRIENT ANALYSIS FOR ONE SERVING

Calories 415	Carbohydrates 66 g	Total Fat 13 g
Protein 10 g	**Fibre** 7 g	**Saturated Fat** 1 g
Sodium 500 mg	**Sugars** 5 g	**Monounsaturated Fat** 7 g
Cholesterol 0 mg		**Polyunsaturated Fat** 3 g

WHITE BEAN STEW

SERVES 4

In this robust stew, rosemary melds perfectly with garlic, black olives, tomatoes, and a touch of dark balsamic vinegar. You can substitute 100 g (4 oz) of dried beans for the tinned beans. (For tips on cooking dried beans, see page 135.)

In a large saucepan, heat the olive oil over medium heat. Add the onion and garlic and sauté about 5 minutes until fragrant. Add the stock and simmer about 5 minutes until the onion is tender. Add the beans, rosemary, salt, and pepper. Simmer, uncovered, for 5 minutes. Add the tomatoes and olives and continue to simmer about 5 minutes longer until the mixture is heated through. Remove from the heat and stir in the vinegar. Ladle into shallow serving bowls and top with the cheese.

2 teaspoons olive oil

1 onion, chopped

4 cloves garlic, crushed

250 ml (8 fl oz) fat-free, no-salt-added chicken or vegetable stock

One 400-g (15-oz) tin no-salt-added haricot or cannellini beans, rinsed and drained

1½ tablespoons chopped fresh rosemary or 1½ teaspoons dried rosemary

¼ teaspoon salt

½ teaspoon freshly ground black pepper

4 large tomatoes or 4 plum tomatoes, seeded and chopped

50 g (2 oz) black olives, sliced and pitted

1 tablespoon balsamic vinegar

15 g (½ oz) grated Romano or Parmesan cheese

NUTRIENT ANALYSIS FOR ONE SERVING

Calories 248	**Carbohydrates** 31 g	**Total Fat** 9 g
Protein 12 g	**Fibre** 10 g	**Saturated Fat** 2 g
Sodium 520 mg	**Sugars** 7 g	**Monounsaturated Fat** 5 g
Cholesterol 7 mg		**Polyunsaturated Fat** 1 g

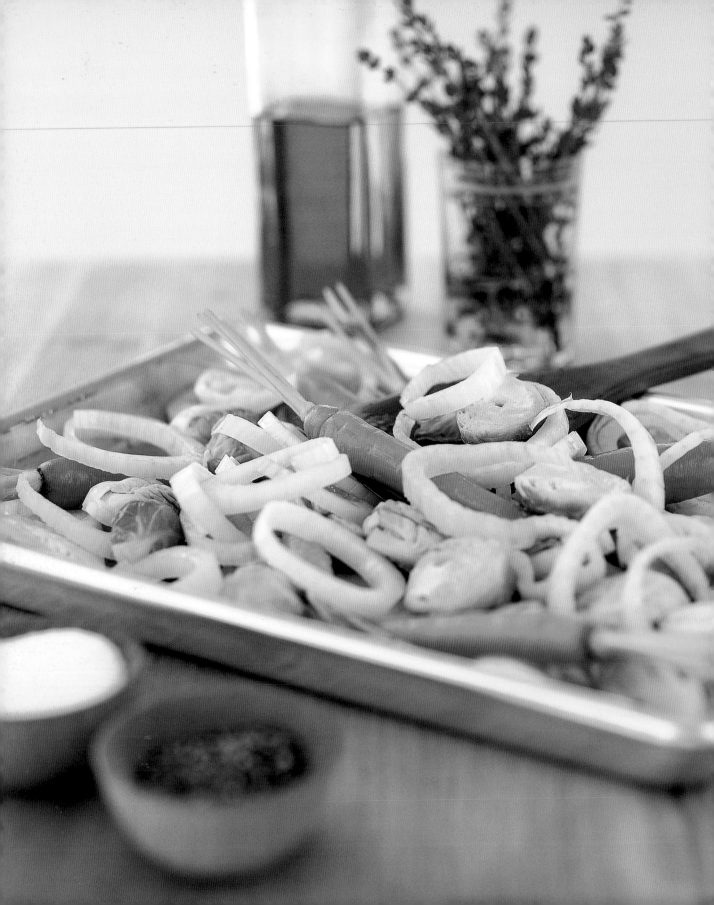

SIDE DISHES

Roasted Winter Vegetables, 115

22g

BLACK-EYED PEAS WITH GREENS

SERVES 6

3 teaspoons olive oil

25 g (1 oz) pancetta (Italian bacon), chopped, or 1 rasher smoked streaky bacon, chopped

½ onion, chopped

½ celery stalk, chopped

2 cloves garlic, crushed

2 x 400-g (15-oz) tins black-eyed peas, rinsed and drained

500 ml (18 fl oz) water

¼ teaspoon salt

50 g (2 oz) spring greens, thickly shredded

2 tablespoons chopped fresh parsley

2 teaspoons red wine vinegar

This classic American dish is flavoured with a small amount of pancetta, or bacon. In addition to being a popular comfort food, the dish is exceptionally healthy – providing fibre, folate, and antioxidants to help protect your heart and blood vessels.

In a large saucepan, heat 1 teaspoon of the olive oil over medium heat. Add the pancetta or bacon and cook 2–3 minutes until lightly browned. Transfer to a plate.

Add the remaining olive oil to the pan and heat over medium heat. Add the onion and celery and sauté for 6–8 minutes, until the vegetables are tender. Stir in the garlic and cook for 1 minute. Add the black-eyed peas, water, salt, and greens. Bring to a boil, reduce the heat to low, and simmer, covered, for 6–8 minutes until the greens wilt and soften. Remove from the heat and stir in the parsley and vinegar.

To serve, ladle into a warmed serving bowl and sprinkle with the browned pancetta or bacon. Serve immediately.

NUTRIENT ANALYSIS FOR ONE SERVING

Calories 146	**Carbohydrates** 22 g	**Total Fat** 3 g
Protein 8 g	**Fibre** 6 g	**Saturated Fat** 1 g
Sodium 129 mg	**Sugars** 4 g	**Monounsaturated Fat** 2 g
Cholesterol 1 mg		**Polyunsaturated Fat** <1 g

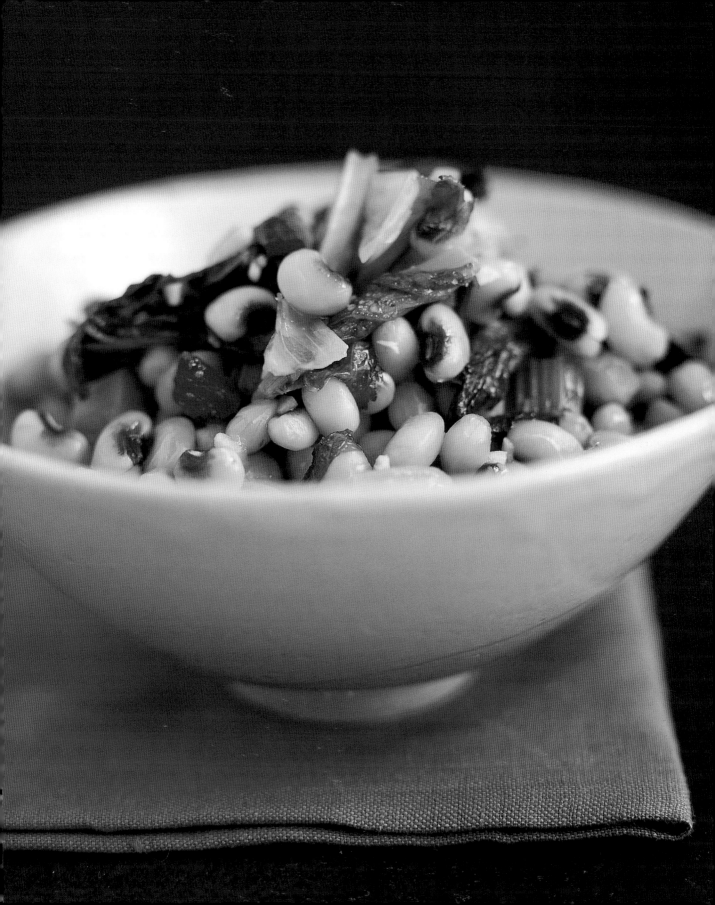

HERBED CHICKPEA RICE

SERVES 6

75 g (3 oz) long-grain brown rice

250 ml (8 fl oz) water

1 bay leaf

⅛ teaspoon salt, plus ¼ teaspoon

One 400-g (15-oz) tin no-salt-added
  chickpeas, rinsed and drained

¼ teaspoon grated lemon zest

1 tablespoon fresh lemon juice

2 teaspoons olive oil

2 tablespoons chopped fresh
  parsley

2 tablespoons chopped fresh basil

1 tablespoon chopped fresh thyme

¼ teaspoon freshly ground black
  pepper

Lemon flavours enliven this tasty, fibre-rich side dish. For a colourful vegetarian meal, pair it with Beetroot & Spinach Salad (page 50). You can substitute 100 g (4 oz) dried haricot beans for the tinned beans. (For tips on cooking dried beans, see page 135.)

In a large saucepan, combine the rice, water, bay leaf, and ⅛ teaspoon of the salt over high heat. Bring the mixture to a boil. Reduce the heat to low, cover, and simmer about 45 minutes until the rice is tender. Add the chickpeas and continue cooking 3–4 minutes until the chickpeas are heated through. Remove from the heat and stir in the lemon zest, the remaining salt, the lemon juice, olive oil, parsley, basil, thyme, and pepper. Serve immediately.

NUTRIENT ANALYSIS FOR ONE SERVING

Calories 157	**Carbohydrates** 27 g	**Total Fat** 3 g
Protein 6 g	**Fibre** 4 g	**Saturated Fat** 0 g
Sodium 154 mg	**Sugars** 3 g	**Monounsaturated Fat** 1 g
Cholesterol 0 mg		**Polyunsaturated Fat** 0 g

SESAME BROCCOLI

CARB COUNT

5g

DIABETIC EXCHANGES

| 0 starch | 0 fruit | 0 milk |
| 1 vegetable | 0 protein | ½ fat |

SERVES 4

Quick, easy, and pretty on the plate, this side dish pairs well with Asian dishes. Try it with Szechuan Pork Stir-Fry (page 76) or Teriyaki Scallops (page 60). Look for sesame seeds in your supermarket's spice rack or at a health-food store.

Put the sesame seeds in a small, dry non-stick frying pan over medium-high heat. Cook for 3–5 minutes, stirring often, until lightly toasted. Set aside.

In a large pot fitted with a steamer basket, bring 2.5 cm (1 in) of water to a boil. Add the broccoli, cover, and steam 7–9 minutes until the stalks are tender. Transfer to a serving bowl. Toss with the soy sauce, sesame oil, and pepper. Garnish with the toasted sesame seeds. Serve immediately.

1 tablespoon sesame seeds

450 g (1 lb) broccoli, trimmed and cut into florets, or 350 g (12 oz) pre-cut fresh broccoli florets or frozen broccoli florets

4 teaspoons low-sodium soy sauce

1 teaspoon dark sesame oil

¼ teaspoon freshly ground black pepper

NUTRIENT ANALYSIS FOR ONE SERVING

Calories 46	**Carbohydrates** 5 g	**Total Fat** 3 g
Protein 3 g	**Fibre** 2 g	**Saturated Fat** 0 g
Sodium 197 mg	**Sugars** 1 g	**Monounsaturated Fat** 1 g
Cholesterol 0 mg		**Polyunsaturated Fat** 1 g

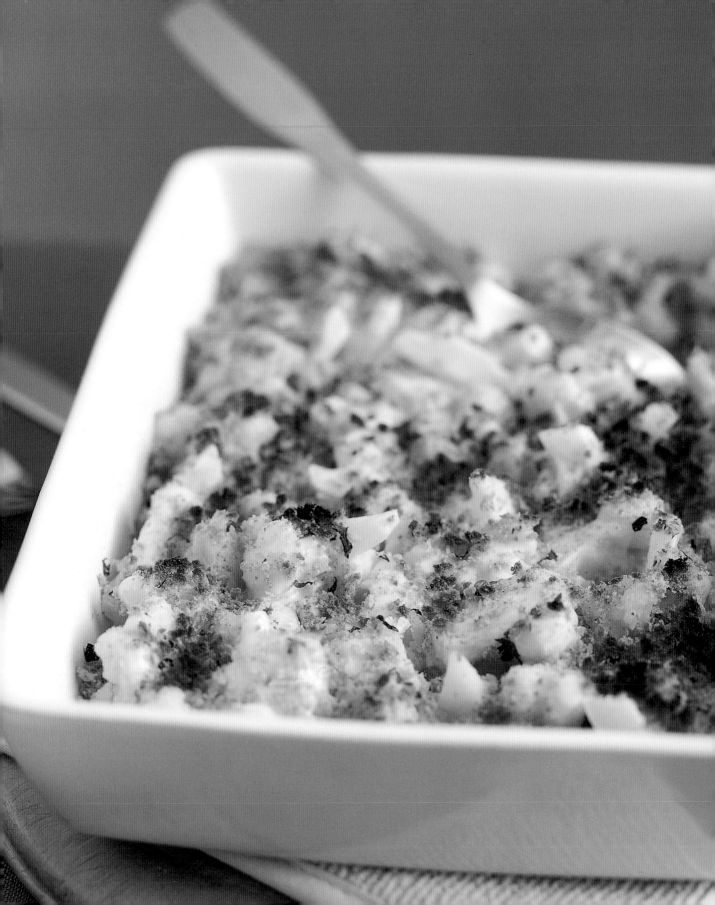

CAULIFLOWER GRATIN

CARB COUNT 13g

DIABETIC EXCHANGES
½ starch   0 fruit   0 milk
1 vegetable   ½ protein   ½ fat

SERVES 4

Topped with seasoned breadcrumbs, this gratin, or French-style casserole, is an elegant dish suitable for guests, yet it is easy to make. The cauliflower is coated with a low-fat cheese sauce, then the dish is baked until browned and bubbly.

Preheat the oven to 200°C (400°F).

In a large pot fitted with a steamer basket, bring 2.5 cm (1 in) of water to a boil. Add the cauliflower, cover, and steam 7–8 minutes until tender. Drain and keep warm.

In a saucepan over medium heat, combine the flour, milk, and nutmeg and whisk to blend. Cook 8–10 minutes until thickened, stirring frequently at first and then constantly as the sauce begins to thicken. Remove from the heat and stir in the cheese, chives, and pepper.

Lightly coat the bottom and sides of a 1¼-litres (2-pt) gratin dish or shallow baking dish with ½ teaspoon of the olive oil. Spoon the cauliflower into the dish, then pour the cheese sauce over.

Place the bread in a small food processor or blender and pulse to form coarse crumbs. Add the parsley and the remaining olive oil and pulse to blend. Sprinkle the breadcrumb mixture evenly over the cauliflower-cheese sauce mixture. Bake about 15 minutes, until the mixture is bubbly and the breadcrumbs are lightly browned. Serve immediately.

350 g (12 oz) cauliflower florets

3 tablespoons plain flour

350 g (12 fl oz) skimmed milk

⅛ teaspoon freshly grated nutmeg

50 g (2 oz) fontina or low-fat Cheddar cheese, grated

1 tablespoon chopped fresh chives

⅛ teaspoon freshly ground black pepper

2 teaspoons olive oil

2 slices wholemeal or multigrain bread, 25 g (1 oz) each, torn into large pieces

1 tablespoon chopped fresh parsley

NUTRIENT ANALYSIS FOR ONE SERVING

Calories 109	**Carbohydrates** 13 g	**Total Fat** 4 g
Protein 6 g	**Fibre** 3 g	**Saturated Fat** 1 g
Sodium 144 mg	**Sugars** 5 g	**Monounsaturated Fat** 1 g
Cholesterol 7 mg		**Polyunsaturated Fat** 0 g

SOYA BEAN SUCCOTASH

SERVES 4

225 g (8 oz) fresh or thawed frozen soya beans, or baby broad beans

10 g (4 oz) butternut squash, peeled and coarsely chopped

1 rasher streaky bacon

½ small onion, chopped

175 g (6 oz) fresh sweetcorn kernels, cut from 1 ear of sweetcorn

2 tablespoons chopped fresh parsley

¼ teaspoon salt

⅛ teaspoon freshly ground black pepper

Fresh soya beans, also called edamame, taste a bit like fresh garden peas. If you wish, you can use baby broad beans instead. Serve with Pork Loin with Apples (page 74) or Polenta-Crusted Haddock Fillets (page 57).

In a small pot fitted with a steamer basket, bring 2.5 cm (1 in) of water to a boil. Add the beans and squash, cover, and steam for 5–6 minutes, until nearly tender. Remove from the heat, drain, and set aside.

In a large non-stick frying pan, cook the bacon over medium heat 2–3 minutes until lightly browned. Transfer the bacon to a paper towel to drain.

With a clean paper towel, wipe the frying pan. Add the onion and sweetcorn to the pan and cook over medium heat about 5 minutes until tender. Add the bean mixture and continue cooking 2–3 minutes longer until the vegetables are warmed through. Remove from the heat. Chop the bacon and stir into the bean mixture along with the parsley, salt, and pepper. Serve immediately.

NUTRIENT ANALYSIS FOR ONE SERVING

Calories 113	Carbohydrates 16 g	Total Fat 4 g
Protein 7 g	Fibre 4 g	Saturated Fat 1 g
Sodium 193 mg	Sugars 1 g	Monounsaturated Fat 1 g
Cholesterol 2 mg		Polyunsaturated Fat 2 g

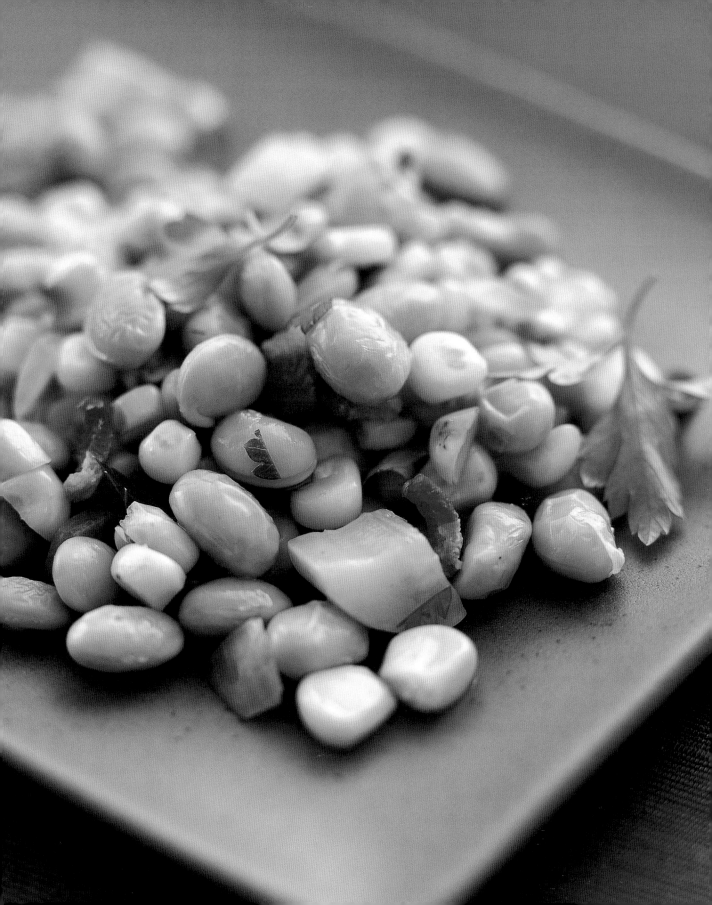

POLENTA WITH GARLIC & BASIL

SERVES 6

1 teaspoon olive oil

2 large cloves garlic, crushed

750 ml (1¼ pt) fat-free,
   no-salt-added chicken stock

250 ml (8 fl oz) water

150 g (5 oz) coarse polenta

⅛ teaspoon salt

25 g (1 oz) fresh basil, chopped

25 g (1 oz) grated Parmesan cheese

A coarse grind of polenta cooked simply in stock, this is delicious with fresh basil and Parmesan cheese. For the best flavour, use freshly grated Parmigiano-Reggiano from Italy. Leftovers can be cut into wedges and grilled or pan seared.

In a saucepan, heat the olive oil over medium-high heat. Add the garlic and sauté about 2 minutes until soft and fragrant. Add the stock and water. Gradually add the polenta, whisking constantly to avoid lumps. Bring the mixture to a boil, whisking frequently. Reduce the heat to low and simmer 15–20 minutes, uncovered, whisking frequently, until the mixture is very thick. Remove from the heat, stir in the salt, basil, and cheese, and serve.

NUTRIENT ANALYSIS FOR ONE SERVING

Calories 145	Carbohydrates 25 g	Total Fat 2 g
Protein 7 g	Fibre 3 g	Saturated Fat 1 g
Sodium 196 mg	Sugars 0 g	Monounsaturated Fat 1 g
Cholesterol 3 mg		Polyunsaturated Fat 0 g

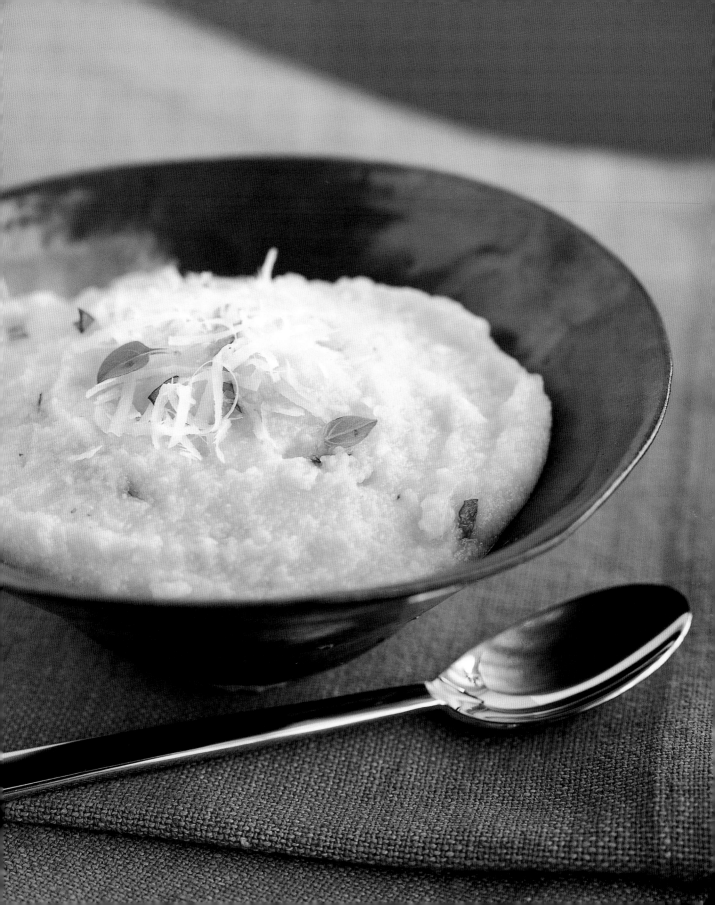

8 g

SAUTÉED WINTER GREENS

SERVES 4

225 g (8 oz) kale, about 14 large leaves

225 g (8 oz) fresh spring greens

225 g (8 oz) red or green Swiss chard

1½ teaspoons olive oil

3 cloves garlic, crushed

⅛ teaspoon salt

⅛ teaspoon freshly ground black pepper

1 tablespoon balsamic or red wine vinegar

Don't be surprised by the amount of chopped kale, greens, and Swiss chard in this recipe – fresh greens cook down greatly. All it takes to finish this quick and tasty dish is a sprinkling of salt and pepper and a splash of mildly sweet balsamic vinegar. Despite the name, spring greens are available all year and are most popular in the winter.

Remove the tough stems and ribs of the kale and discard. Coarsely chop the kale greens and set them aside. Remove the tough stems and ribs of the spring greens and Swiss chard and discard. Coarsely chop the spring greens and then the Swiss chard greens, keeping them separate from each other and from the chopped kale.

In a large pot fitted with a steamer basket, bring 2.5 cm (1 in) of water to a boil. Spread the kale in a single layer on the bottom; top with the spring greens and then the Swiss chard. Cover and steam about 10 minutes until the greens are tender. Drain and set aside.

In a large non-stick frying pan, heat the olive oil over medium heat. Stir in the garlic and sauté for 45–60 seconds until it just begins to brown. Add the steamed greens and sauté until the liquid is completely evaporated. Remove from the heat and stir in the salt, pepper, and vinegar. Serve immediately.

NUTRIENT ANALYSIS FOR ONE SERVING

Calories 55	**Carbohydrates** 8 g	**Total Fat** 2 g
Protein 3 g	**Fibre** 3 g	**Saturated Fat** 0 g
Sodium 200 mg	**Sugars** 2 g	**Monounsaturated Fat** 1 g
Cholesterol 0 mg		**Polyunsaturated Fat** 0 g

MASHED SWEET POTATOES

CARB COUNT 22g

DIABETIC EXCHANGES

| 1½ starch | 0 fruit | 0 milk |
| 0 vegetable | 0 protein | ½ fat |

SERVES 4

Sweet potatoes – with all the comfort-food qualities of regular potatoes plus a dose of healthful beta-carotene – deserve to find their way into more dinners. Sprinkled with toasted pecans, these seasoned potatoes pair perfectly with roasted chicken.

Place the sweet potatoes in a saucepan and add water to cover the potatoes. Cover and bring to a boil over high heat. Reduce the heat to low and simmer 12–14 minutes until the potatoes are tender.

While the sweet potatoes are cooking, put the pecans in a small, dry non-stick frying pan over medium-high heat. Cook 3–5 minutes, stirring often, until lightly toasted. Set aside.

Drain the potatoes in a colander, then return them to the same saucepan over low heat. Add the stock, salt, and nutmeg. Using a potato masher or hand-held blender, mash the potatoes until light and fluffy. Transfer to individual plates and top with the toasted pecans.

450 g (1 lb) sweet potatoes, peeled and cut into 2-cm (¾-in) chunks

2 tablespoons chopped pecans

85 ml (2½ fl oz) fat-free, no-salt-added chicken or vegetable stock

¼ teaspoon salt

⅛ teaspoon freshly grated nutmeg

NUTRIENT ANALYSIS FOR ONE SERVING

Calories 121	Carbohydrates 22 g	Total Fat 3 g
Protein 2 g	Fibre 2 g	Saturated Fat 0 g
Sodium 171 mg	Sugars 10 g	Monounsaturated Fat 2 g
Cholesterol 0 mg		Polyunsaturated Fat 1 g

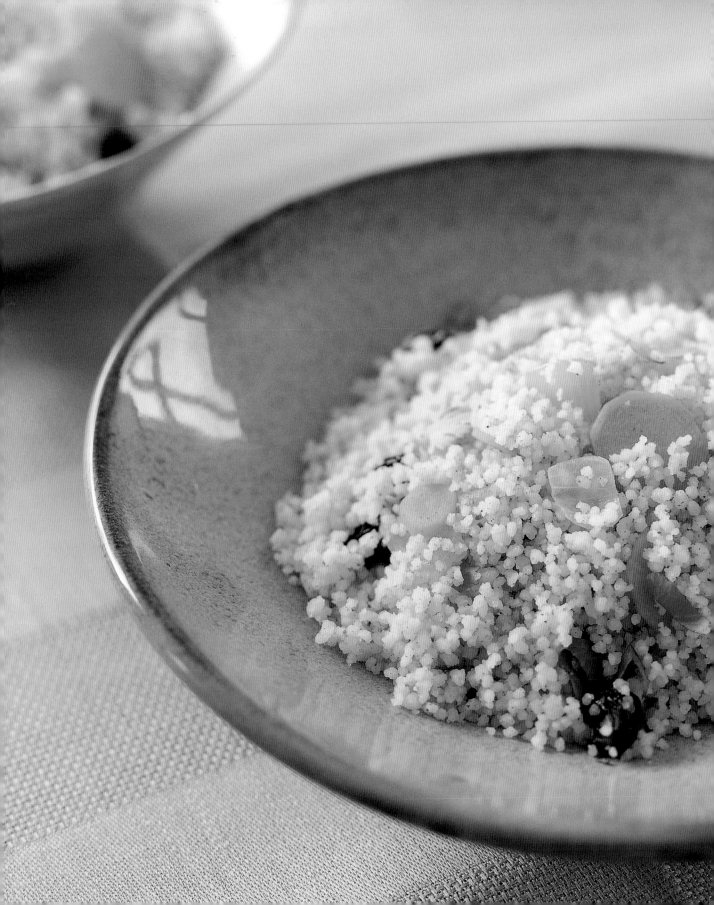

COUSCOUS WITH RAISINS & SPICES

CARB COUNT 28g

DIABETIC EXCHANGES
1½ starch	0 fruit	0 milk
½ vegetable	½ protein	0 fat

SERVES 6

Made like pasta from the hard durum wheat called semolina, couscous is a mild, easy-to-use grain product that cooks in minutes. Vegetables and seasonings now common in supermarkets give this dish its enticing North African flavour.

In a saucepan, heat the olive oil over medium heat. Add the onion, carrot, and garlic and sauté about 5 minutes until fragrant. Add the ground coriander, cumin, and cinnamon to the vegetables and continue to sauté about 1 minute. Add the stock, raisins, and salt and bring to a simmer. Reduce the heat to low and simmer, uncovered, for about 3 minutes until the vegetables are tender. Stir in the couscous. Cover the saucepan and remove it from the heat. Let stand about 5 minutes, until the couscous has absorbed the liquid. Fluff with a fork. Transfer to individual plates and top with the fresh coriander.

1 teaspoon olive oil

1 small onion, chopped

1 small carrot, thinly sliced

3 cloves garlic, crushed

1 teaspoon ground coriander

¾ teaspoon ground cumin

¼ teaspoon ground cinnamon

425 ml (14½ fl oz) fat-free, no-salt-added chicken or vegetable stock

3 tablespoons dark raisins or sultanas

¼ teaspoon salt

100 g (4 oz) couscous or wholewheat couscous

2 tablespoons chopped fresh coriander

NUTRIENT ANALYSIS FOR ONE SERVING

Calories 149	**Carbohydrates** 28 g	**Total Fat** 1 g
Protein 6 g	**Fibre** 3 g	**Saturated Fat** 0 g
Sodium 156 mg	**Sugars** 5 g	**Monounsaturated Fat** 1 g
Cholesterol 0 mg		**Polyunsaturated Fat** 0 g

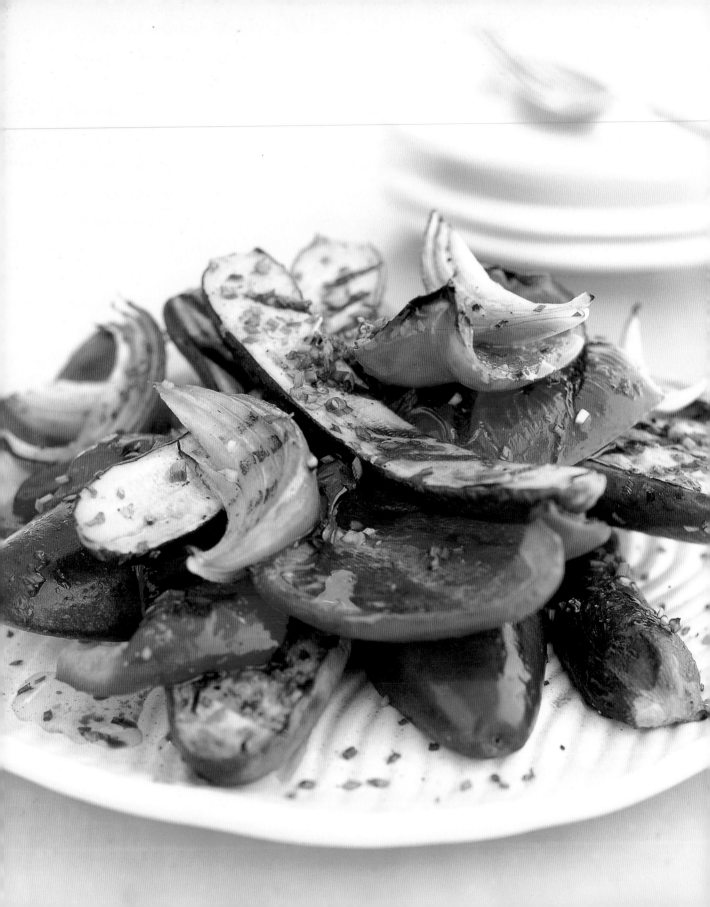

GRILLED SUMMER VEGETABLES

CARB COUNT 15g

DIABETIC EXCHANGES
| ½ starch | 0 fruit | 0 milk |
| 2 vegetable | 0 protein | ½ fat |

SERVES 4

This colourful dish takes full advantage of summer's bounty of squash, sweet peppers, and aubergines. Brushed with vinaigrette and grilled, the vegetables take on a pleasing smokiness that makes them a fine accompaniment for grilled chicken or salmon. A ridged griddle pan can also be used to cook this dish. Cook in batches and keep warm.

Preheat a grill or prepare a barbecue. Position the cooking rack 10–15 cm (4–6 in) from the heat source.

In a small bowl, combine the stock, vinegar, olive oil, garlic, salt, and black pepper. Brush half of the stock mixture over the aubergines, sweet peppers, courgettes, and onion. Place the vegetables on the grill rack. Grill for about 6 minutes, until the vegetables begin to brown. Turn the vegetables over and brush with the remaining stock mixture. Continue cooking about 5 minutes longer until the vegetables are lightly browned and tender-crisp. Transfer to a platter and top with the basil.

- 4 tablespoons fat-free, no-salt-added chicken or vegetable stock
- 1 tablespoon balsamic vinegar
- 2 teaspoons olive oil
- 2 cloves garlic, crushed
- ¼ teaspoon salt
- ¼ teaspoon freshly ground black pepper
- 2 Asian aubergines, halved lengthwise
- 2 red or yellow sweet peppers, or 1 of each, seeded and cut lengthwise into quarters
- 2 courgettes, halved lengthwise
- 1 small red onion, cut into slices 6 mm (¼ in) thick
- 2 tablespoons chopped fresh basil or chives

NUTRIENT ANALYSIS FOR ONE SERVING

Calories 88	Carbohydrates 15 g	Total Fat 3 g
Protein 4 g	Fibre 5 g	Saturated Fat 0 g
Sodium 165 mg	Sugars 8 g	Monounsaturated Fat 2 g
Cholesterol 0 mg		Polyunsaturated Fat 0 g

8g

GREEN BEANS WITH TOMATOES & GARLIC

SERVES 4

- 450 g (1 lb) green beans
- 3–4 tomatoes, seeded and chopped
- 1 tablespoon capers, rinsed
- 1½ teaspoons olive oil
- 1 clove garlic, crushed
- ⅛ teaspoon salt
- 1 anchovy fillet, mashed, or ½ teaspoon anchovy paste (optional)

The sweetness of green beans melds wonderfully with the traditional French blend of tomatoes, olive oil, garlic, and capers. To make this dish even more authentic, use delicate, thin French green beans.

Place the green beans in a frying pan or saucepan and add water to cover. Bring to a boil over high heat. Reduce the heat to low and simmer, uncovered, 4–6 minutes until tender, depending on the beans' thickness. Drain.

While the beans are cooking, in a bowl, combine the tomatoes, capers, olive oil, garlic, and salt and stir to mix. Stir in the anchovy, if using.

Transfer the cooked beans to a serving bowl, add the tomato mixture, and toss to mix. Serve immediately.

NUTRIENT ANALYSIS FOR ONE SERVING

Calories 55	Carbohydrates 8 g	Total Fat 2 g
Protein 1 g	Fibre 4 g	Saturated Fat 0 g
Sodium 139 mg	Sugars 3 g	Monounsaturated Fat 1 g
Cholesterol 0 mg		Polyunsaturated Fat 0 g

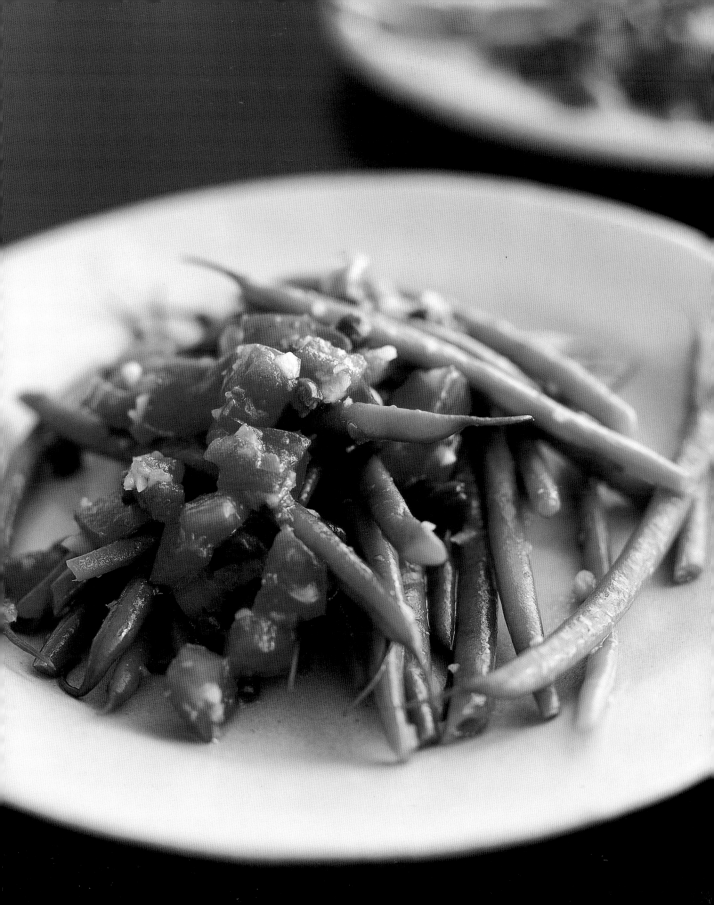

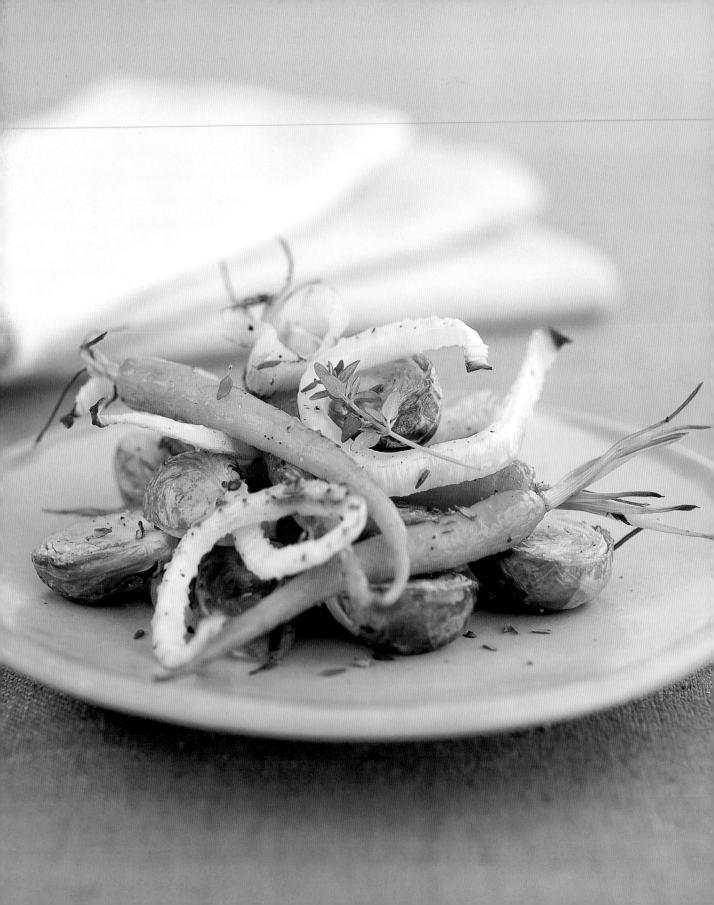

ROASTED WINTER VEGETABLES

SERVES 4

CARB COUNT 14g

DIABETIC EXCHANGES
| 0 starch | 0 fruit | 0 milk |
| 2½ vegetable | 0 protein | ½ fat |

It's now easy to find once-exotic items such as fennel bulbs. The feathery tops resemble fresh dill and can be used like any fresh herb. Similar in texture to celery, fennel bulb has a subtle anise flavour that goes well in this mix of roasted vegetables.

Preheat the oven to 190°C (375°F).

Trim the ends of the fennel bulb and cut the bulb through the core into 6-mm (¼-in) slices. Cut each brussels sprout through the core into halves. Combine the fennel, brussels sprouts, and carrots in a shallow roasting pan or rimmed baking sheet. Sprinkle the vegetables with the olive oil, salt, and pepper and toss to coat. Roast for about 30 minutes, until the vegetables are tender. Sprinkle the vegetables with the chopped fennel fronds and the thyme, if desired.

- 1 large fennel bulb, about 225 g (8 oz), green fronds reserved for garnish (about 2 tablespoons chopped)
- 225 g (8 oz) brussels sprouts
- 225 g (8 oz) baby carrots
- 2 teaspoons olive oil
- ⅛ teaspoon salt
- ¼ teaspoon freshly ground black pepper
- 1 tablespoon chopped fresh thyme (optional)

NUTRIENT ANALYSIS FOR ONE SERVING

Calories 82	Carbohydrates 14 g	Total Fat 3 g
Protein 3 g	Fibre 5 g	Saturated Fat 0 g
Sodium 136 mg	Sugars 4 g	Monounsaturated Fat 2 g
Cholesterol 0 mg		Polyunsaturated Fat 0 g

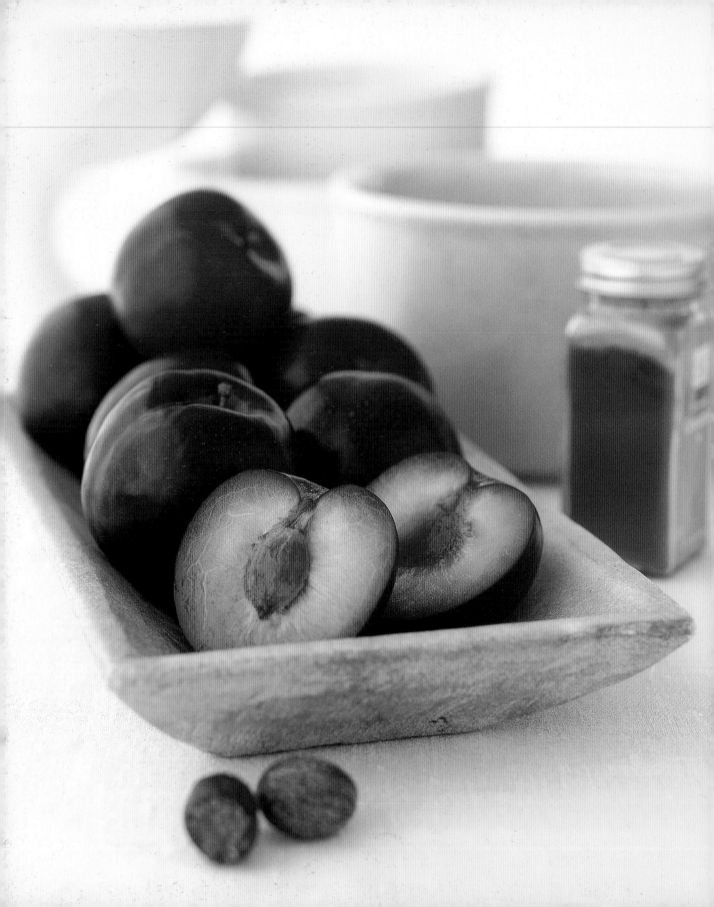

DESSERTS & SNACKS

APPLE CRISP

SERVES 5

4 tablespoons unsweetened apple juice

2 teaspoons cornflour

6 medium Bramley cooking apples, peeled, cored, and sliced

1 tablespoon almond-flavoured liqueur, such as amaretto (optional)

1½ teaspoons ground cinnamon

50 g (2 oz) old-fashioned rolled oats

1 tablespoon sunflower oil

40 g (1½ oz) firmly packed light brown sugar

2 tablespoons chopped walnuts

This quick fruit crisp, made with walnuts and a small amount of healthy sunflower oil, is every bit as richly satisfying as apple crumble, without any of the unhealthy saturated and trans fats. Granny Smith apples can also be used in this recipe.

Preheat the oven to 190°C (375°F).

In a bowl, combine the apple juice and cornflour and stir until the cornflour dissolves. Add the apples, the liqueur (if using), and 1 teaspoon of the cinnamon and toss well to mix. Transfer the mixture to a 20-cm (8-in) square baking dish or a deep 23-cm (9-in) pie dish.

In a bowl, combine the oats and sunflower oil and mix well. Add the brown sugar, walnuts, and the remaining cinnamon. Sprinkle the mixture over the apples. Bake 35–40 minutes until the apples are tender and the topping is golden brown. Serve warm or at room temperature.

NUTRIENT ANALYSIS FOR ONE SERVING

Calories 180	Carbohydrates 34 g	Total Fat 6 g
Protein 1 g	**Fibre** 3 g	**Saturated Fat** 0 g
Sodium 6 mg	**Sugars** 26 g	**Monounsaturated Fat** 2 g
Cholesterol 0 mg		**Polyunsaturated Fat** 2 g

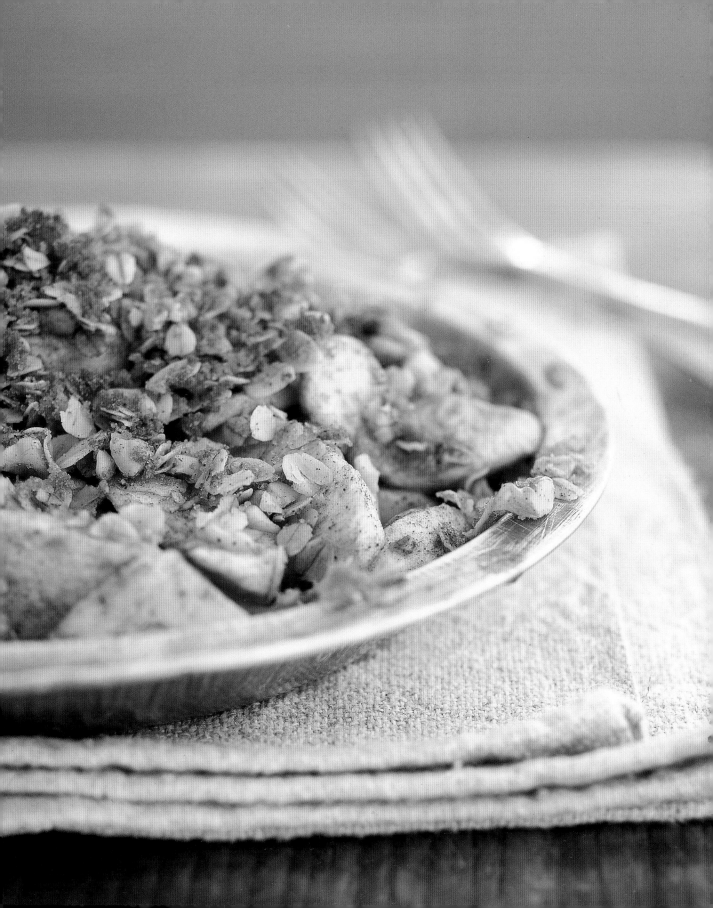

DIABETIC EXCHANGES

0 starch	1 fruit	0 milk
0 vegetable	0 protein	½ fat

ROASTED PLUMS

SERVES 4

2 tablespoons frozen apple juice concentrate, thawed

⅛ teaspoon ground cinnamon

Pinch of freshly grated nutmeg

6–8 plums, about 450 g (1 lb) total weight, cut in half and stoned

1 teaspoon sunflower oil

4 teaspoons cream sherry (optional)

2 teaspoons chopped pistachios

Both sweet and tart by nature, plums are the ideal fruit for this flavourful dessert. Peaches and apricots also lend themselves wonderfully to this preparation, which is reminiscent of baked apples. Top with vanilla yoghurt instead of sherry, if you prefer. If you cannot find apple juice concentrate, reduce 6 tablespoons of unsweetened apple juice in a pan to 2 tablespoons.

Preheat the oven to 230°C (450°F).

In a bowl, combine the apple juice concentrate, cinnamon, and a generous pinch of nutmeg. Add the plums and toss gently to mix.

Lightly coat the bottom of a small baking dish with the sunflower oil. Arrange the plum halves cut sides down in a single layer in the dish. Pour in any of the juice mixture remaining in the bowl. Bake about 15 minutes until the plums are tender and the juice has reduced to a syrup. Drizzle each serving with 1 teaspoon sherry, if desired, and sprinkle with the pistachios. Serve immediately, or let cool to room temperature and serve.

NUTRIENT ANALYSIS FOR ONE SERVING

Calories 101	**Carbohydrates** 18 g	**Total Fat** 3 g
Protein 1 g	**Fibre** 2 g	**Saturated Fat** 0 g
Sodium 2 mg	**Sugars** 10 g	**Monounsaturated Fat** 2 g
Cholesterol 0 mg		**Polyunsaturated Fat** 1 g

PISTACHIO CLOUDS

MAKES 24 BISCUITS

Roasted pistachios and cocoa powder give these crisp biscuits a delightfully rich flavour, while rolled oats add some fibre and egg whites keep them feather light. What's more, they're easy to make. Serve for dessert or as a mid-afternoon snack.

Preheat the oven to 170°C (325°F).

In a bowl, combine the oats, brown sugar, cocoa powder, pistachios, flour, and salt and stir to mix well. Set aside.

In a spotlessly clean, large bowl or the bowl of a stand mixer, beat the egg whites at high speed until soft peaks form. Add the granulated sugar, 1 tablespoon at a time, and the vanilla, beating until stiff peaks form. Gently fold the oat mixture into the beaten egg whites, mixing just until no white streaks remain.

Lightly coat 2 baking sheets with cooking spray. With a soup spoon, drop the dough onto the baking sheets in rounded spoonfuls, spaced 2.5 cm (1 in) apart. Bake 16–18 minutes until set. Let the biscuits cool on the baking sheets for 1 minute. With a palette knife, transfer the biscuits to cooling racks and let cool completely. Store tightly covered at room temperature for up to 2 days or freeze for up to 2 weeks.

40 g (1½ oz) quick-cooking rolled oats

50 g (2 oz) firmly packed light brown sugar

40 g (1½ oz) unsweetened cocoa powder

40 g (1½ oz) pistachios or pecans, chopped and toasted (page 138)

2 tablespoons plain flour

¼ teaspoon salt

4 egg whites

4 tablespoons granulated sugar

1 teaspoon vanilla extract

Cooking spray

NUTRIENT ANALYSIS FOR ONE BISCUIT

Calories 47	**Carbohydrates** 8 g	**Total Fat** 1 g
Protein 2 g	**Fibre** 1 g	**Saturated Fat** 0 g
Sodium 35 mg	**Sugars** 5 g	**Monounsaturated Fat** 1 g
Cholesterol 0 mg		**Polyunsaturated Fat** 0 g

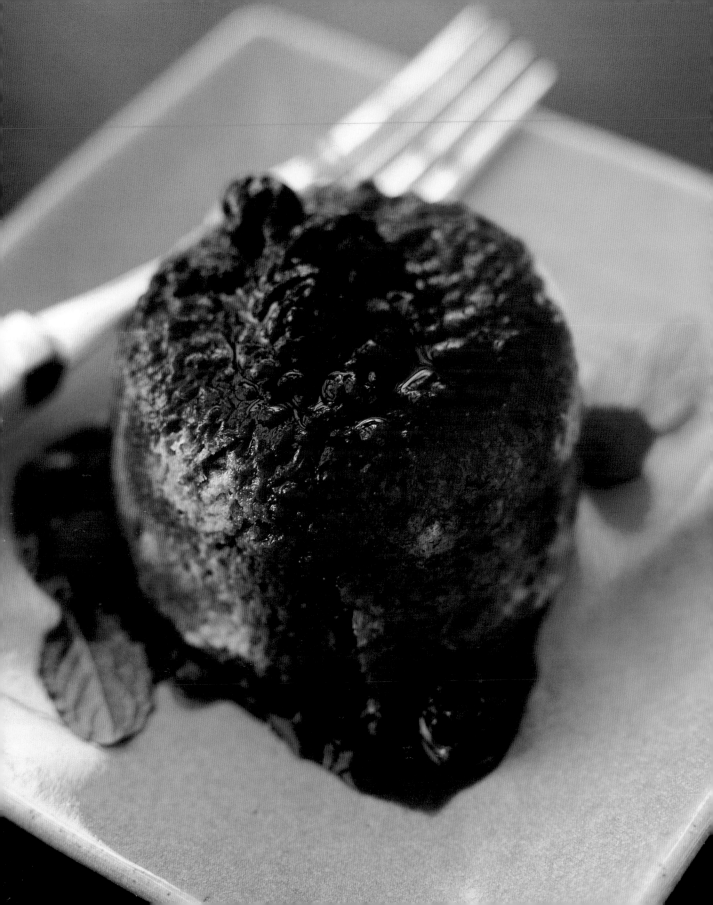

MIXED BERRY SUMMER PUDDING

CARB COUNT 41g

DIABETIC EXCHANGES

| 1 starch | 1 fruit | 0 milk |
| 0 vegetable | 0 protein | 0 fat |

SERVES 4

This venerable dessert is one of Britain's traditional puddings. It's very easy to make: tangy ripe berries sandwiched in juice-sweetened bread, then refrigerated until the ingredients gel.

In a small saucepan, combine the blueberries, blackberries, raspberries, orange zest, and orange juice. Bring the mixture to a boil over medium-high heat. Cook at a gentle boil for 2 minutes. Remove from the heat and stir in the jam. Set aside.

Using a 10-g (4-oz) ramekin as a guide, cut a round from 4 of the bread slices to fit into the bottom of each of the 4 ramekins. Slice the bread scraps to fit the sides of the ramekins and tuck in to fit. Carefully spoon one-quarter of the berry mixture into each ramekin, reserving any extra juice. Cut the remaining 2 bread slices to make rounds that fit into the top of the ramekins. Discard the remaining bread scraps. Press the bread gently with your fingers so it absorbs the juice from the berries. Cover each ramekin with cling film and refrigerate until ready to serve, up to 8 hours.

To serve, place a small dessert plate over the top of each ramekin, invert the plate and ramekin together, and shake gently to transfer the pudding to the plate. Top with the reserved juice and garnish with a mint leaf and blackberries. Serve immediately.

150 g (5 oz) fresh blueberries or frozen blueberries, thawed

150 g (5 oz) fresh blackberries or frozen blackberries, thawed, plus extra berries for garnish

150 g (5 oz) fresh raspberries or frozen raspberries, thawed

½ teaspoon grated orange zest

90 ml (3 fl oz) orange juice

2 tablespoons seedless all-fruit raspberry or blueberry jam

6 thin slices firm, wholemeal bread, crusts removed

Fresh mint leaves for garnish

NUTRIENT ANALYSIS FOR ONE SERVING

Calories 191	Carbohydrates 41 g	Total Fat 2 g
Protein 5 g	Fibre 8 g	Saturated Fat 0 g
Sodium 199 mg	Sugars 19 g	Monounsaturated Fat 1 g
Cholesterol 0 mg		Polyunsaturated Fat 1 g

MANGO-LIME SORBET

DIABETIC EXCHANGES

| 0 starch | 1 fruit | 0 milk |
| 0 vegetable | 0 protein | 0 fat |

SERVES 4

175 ml (6 fl oz) white grape juice

2 large mangoes, about 700 g
    (1½ lb) total weight, peeled and
    coarsely chopped

125 ml (4 fl oz) skimmed milk

1½ teaspoons grated lime zest

4 tablespoons fresh lime juice

Ripe mangoes are so sweet and flavourful they can be puréed into a sensational sorbet with just a touch of added sugar – or, as in this recipe, grape juice. Perfectly ripe mangoes are mildly fragrant and slightly soft to the touch.

Place the grape juice in a small pan and bring to the boil. Boil rapidly until reduced by two-thirds. Allow to cool.

In a food processor, combine the mangoes, reduced grape juice, milk, lime zest, and lime juice and process until smooth. Pour the mango mixture into a glass measuring cup or bowl and chill in the refrigerator for at least 2 hours.

Pour the chilled mango mixture into an ice-cream maker and freeze according to the manufacturer's directions. Serve immediately, or spoon the sorbet into a freezer-safe container and freeze until ready to serve.

NUTRIENT ANALYSIS FOR ONE SERVING

Calories 86	Carbohydrates 21 g	Total Fat 0 g
Protein 1 g	Fibre 2 g	Saturated Fat 0 g
Sodium 19 mg	Sugars 19 g	Monounsaturated Fat 0 g
Cholesterol 0 mg		Polyunsaturated Fat 0 g

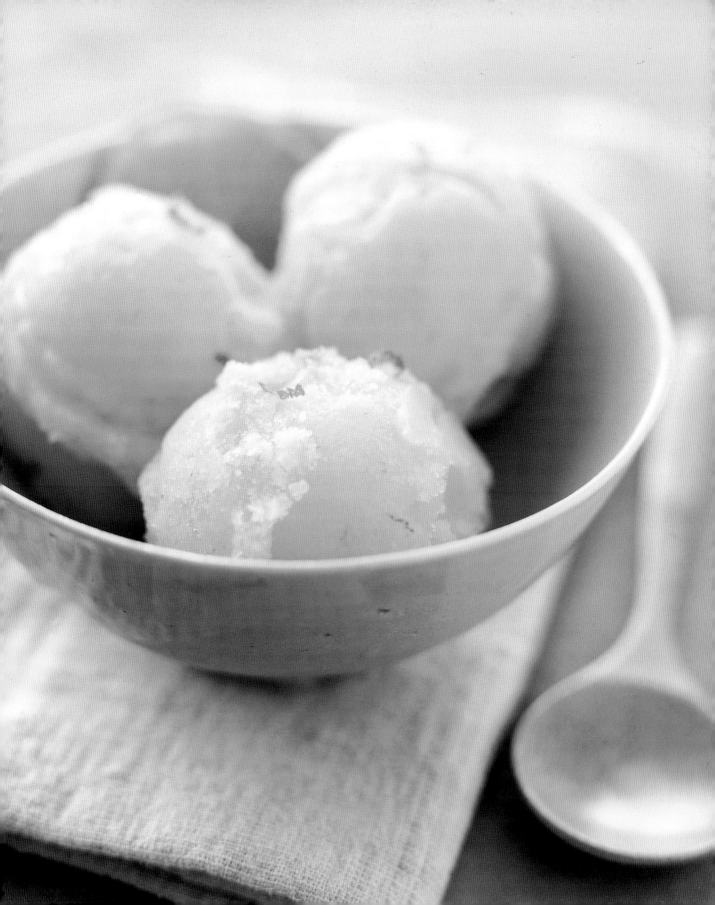

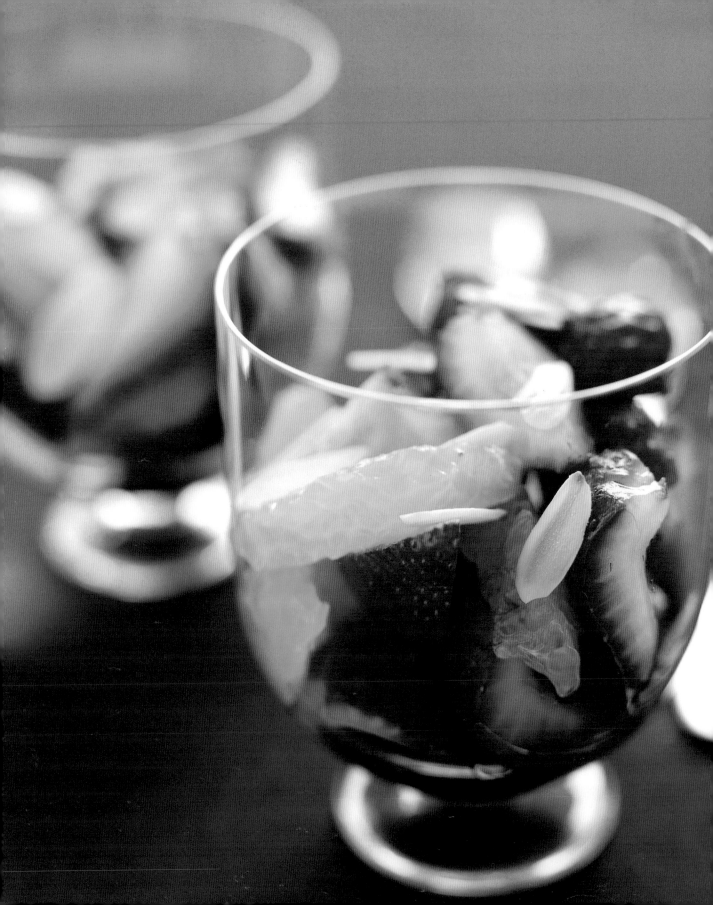

BALSAMIC-GLAZED BERRIES & TANGERINES

CARB COUNT 25g

DIABETIC EXCHANGES

| 0 starch | 1 fruit | ½ other carbs |
| 0 vegetable | 0 protein | ½ fat |

SERVES 4

This elegant and delicious dessert takes just minutes to prepare. For an alternate sauce, combine 2 tablespoons peach or apricot jam (remove large fruit pieces) with 1 tablespoon white wine vinegar. Spoon over the fruit and sprinkle with almonds.

Cut the tangerine segments in half crosswise and combine them with the sliced strawberries in small individual bowls, dividing evenly. In a small saucepan over medium heat, combine the vinegar and brown sugar. Bring to a simmer and cook, uncovered, for 1 minute, stirring frequently. Remove the pan from the heat and let stand for 1–2 minutes until the glaze thickens. Spoon the glaze over the fruit and top with the almonds.

4 tangerines or clementines, peeled and separated into segments

225 g (8 oz) sliced strawberries

2 tablespoons balsamic vinegar

2 tablespoons firmly packed light brown sugar

3 tablespoons flaked almonds, toasted

NUTRIENT ANALYSIS FOR ONE SERVING

Calories 125	**Carbohydrates** 25 g	**Total Fat** 3 g
Protein 2 g	**Fibre** 5 g	**Saturated Fat** 0 g
Sodium 6 mg	**Sugars** 21 g	**Monounsaturated Fat** 1 g
Cholesterol 0 mg		**Polyunsaturated Fat** 1 g

PINEAPPLE SMOOTHIE

SERVES 2

1 small banana, about 150 g (5 oz), cut into 2.5-cm (1-in) chunks

1 tablespoon unsweetened desiccated coconut

200 g (7 oz) fresh pineapple chunks, plus diced pineapple for garnish

125 ml (4 fl oz) low-fat plain yoghurt

125 ml (4 fl oz) soya milk

4 tablespoons mango nectar or orange juice

2 tablespoons toasted wheat germ

⅛ teaspoon freshly grated nutmeg

The refreshing fruit blends called smoothies are among the simplest and most versatile of snacks. Here, tangy pineapple and ripe banana complement the protein-rich yoghurt and soya milk, while nutty wheat germ adds fibre and nutrients.

Place the banana chunks in a freezer-safe bag or container, transfer to the freezer, and freeze until firm, at least 3 hours.

Place the coconut in a small, dry frying pan over medium heat and cook about 2 minutes, stirring constantly, until lightly toasted. Transfer to a plate and set aside.

In a food processor or blender, combine the frozen banana, pineapple chunks, and yoghurt. Process until smooth. Add the soya milk, mango nectar, wheat germ, and nutmeg. Pulse to blend.

Pour the mixture into two 225-ml (8-fl oz) glasses. Garnish with the diced fresh pineapple and coconut. Serve immediately.

NUTRIENT ANALYSIS FOR ONE SERVING

Calories 197	Carbohydrates 38 g	Total Fat 3 g
Protein 8 g	**Fibre** 4 g	**Saturated Fat** 1 g
Sodium 63 mg	**Sugars** 28 g	**Monounsaturated Fat** 1 g
Cholesterol 1 mg		**Polyunsaturated Fat** 1 g

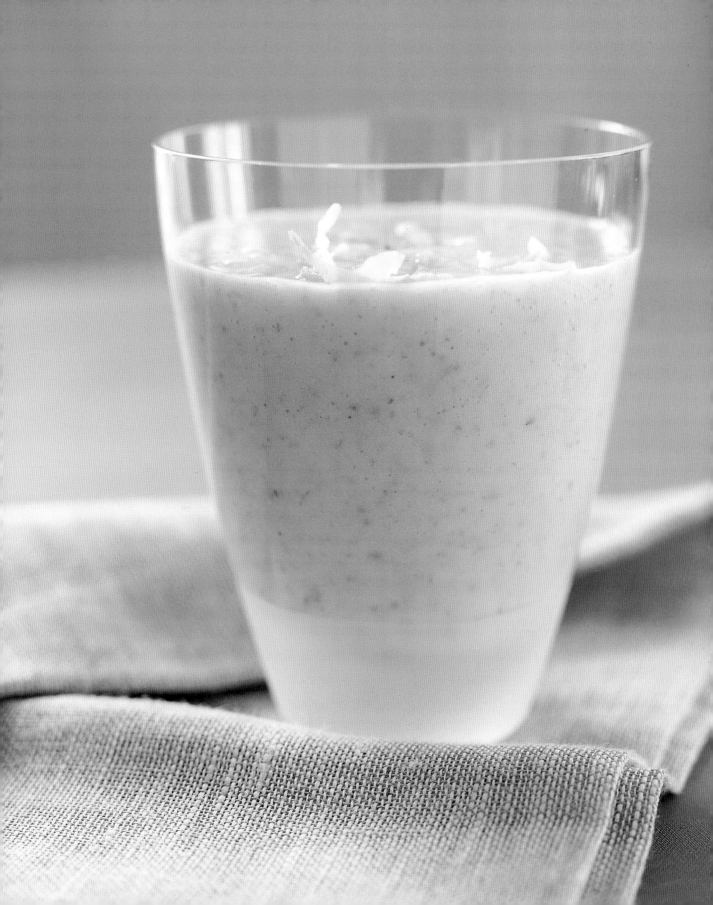

17g

OATMEAL BISCUITS

MAKES 24 BISCUITS

225 g (8 oz) old-fashioned
    rolled oats

100 g (4 oz) plain flour

1 teaspoon baking powder

1½ teaspoons ground cinnamon

¼ teaspoon salt

¼ teaspoon freshly grated nutmeg

90 g (3½ oz) sultanas or
    dark raisins

100 g (4 oz) granulated sugar

4 tablespoons sunflower oil

4 tablespoons unsweetened
    applesauce

4 tablespoons firmly packed light
    brown sugar

1 egg white

1 teaspoon vanilla extract

Moist, chewy, and aromatic with familiar spices, these foolproof cookies made with fibre-rich old-fashioned rolled oats easily qualify as a heart-healthy dessert or snack. For the very best flavour, use freshly grated nutmeg.

Preheat the oven to 180°C (350°F).

In a bowl, combine the oats, flour, baking powder, cinnamon, salt, and nutmeg. In a large bowl, combine the sultanas, granulated sugar, sunflower oil, applesauce, brown sugar, egg white, and vanilla. Stir well to mix. Add the oat mixture to the raisin mixture and stir well to mix.

With a spoon, drop the dough onto 2 ungreased baking sheets in rounded spoonfuls, about 1½ tablespoons each, spaced 5 cm (2 in) apart. Bake 10–12 minutes until the biscuits are firm. Let the biscuits cool on the baking sheets for 2 minutes. With a palette knife, transfer the biscuits to wire cooling racks and let cool completely.

NUTRIENT ANALYSIS FOR ONE BISCUIT

Calories 99	**Carbohydrates** 17 g	**Total Fat** 3 g
Protein 2 g	**Fibre** 1 g	**Saturated Fat** 0 g
Sodium 81 mg	**Sugars** 9 g	**Monounsaturated Fat** 2 g
Cholesterol 0 mg		**Polyunsaturated Fat** 1 g

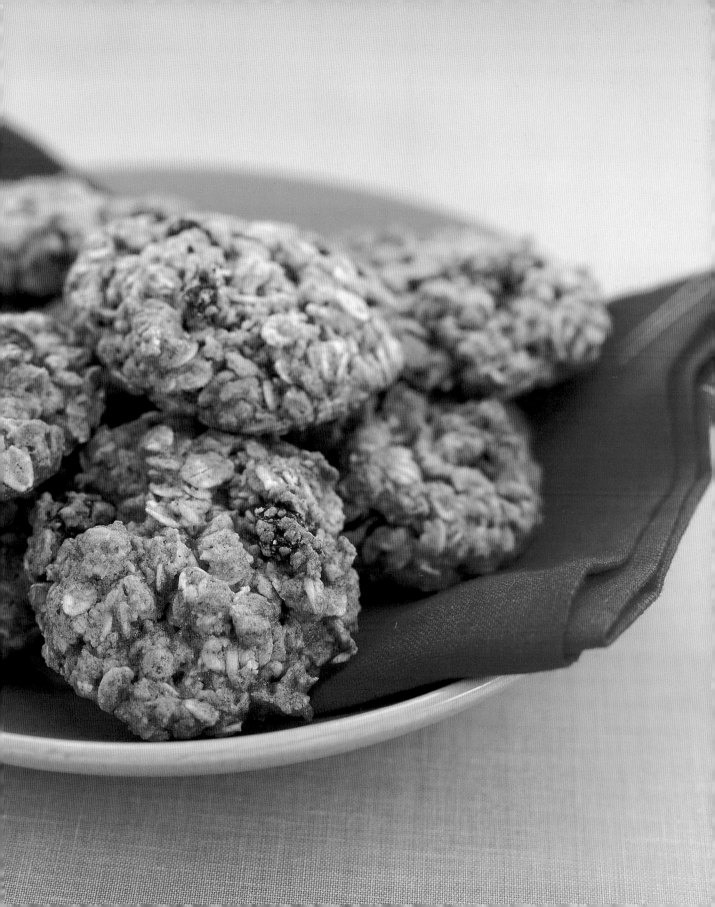

26g

DIABETIC EXCHANGES

1 starch	0 fruit	½ other carbs
0 vegetable	0 protein	1 fat

BLUEBERRY BRAN MUFFINS

MAKES 12 MUFFINS

100 g (4 oz) plain flour

100 g (4 oz) wholemeal flour

100 g (4 oz) wheat bran

3 tablespoons freshly ground linseed or linseed meal

1¼ teaspoons bicarbonate of soda

⅛ teaspoon salt

175 ml (6 fl oz) low-fat buttermilk

125 ml (4 fl oz) low-fat plain yoghurt

2 large eggs, lightly beaten

100 g (4 oz) sugar

3 tablespoons sunflower oil, plus 1 teaspoon

150 g (5 oz) fresh blueberries or frozen blueberries, thawed

The nutty flavour of these supremely light muffins comes from a mix of wholemeal flour, wheat bran, and ground linseed, which is rich in heart-healthy Omega-3 fatty acids. Antioxidant-rich blueberries add a burst of sweetness. You can grind your own seeds in a coffee grinder.

Preheat the oven to 190°C (350°F).

In a large bowl, combine the plain flour, wholemeal flour, wheat bran, ground linseed, bicarbonate of soda, and salt. Whisk to blend.

In another bowl, combine the buttermilk, yoghurt, beaten eggs, sugar, and 3 tablespoons of the sunflower oil. Whisk until well blended. Pour the buttermilk mixture into the flour mixture and stir until just moistened. (Do not overmix the batter or the muffins will be tough.) Fold the blueberries into the batter.

Coat the cups of a 12-cup non-stick muffin pan with the remaining oil, or lightly coat the pan with cooking spray. Spoon the batter into the muffin cups, filling each about two-thirds full. Bake 18–20 minutes until a skewer inserted into the centre of a muffin comes out clean. Cool in the pan on a wire rack for 10 minutes. Remove the muffins from the pan and serve immediately, or let cool on the rack.

NUTRIENT ANALYSIS FOR ONE MUFFIN

Calories 166	**Carbohydrates** 26 g	**Total Fat** 6 g
Protein 5 g	**Fibre** 4 g	**Saturated Fat** 1 g
Sodium 190 mg	**Sugars** 11 g	**Monounsaturated Fat** 3 g
Cholesterol 36 mg		**Polyunsaturated Fat** 2 g

SPICY PITTA CRISPS

CARB COUNT **13**g

DIABETIC EXCHANGES

| 1 starch | 0 fruit | 0 milk |
| 0 vegetable | 0 protein | ½ fat |

SERVES 4

These fibre-rich snacks get an invigorating zing from a dusting of cayenne pepper. For less spicy chips, reduce the amount of cayenne pepper to ⅛ teaspoon. Enjoy the crisps plain, or serve with the Vegetable Platter with Hummus Dip (page 34).

Preheat the oven to 200°C (400°F).

Using a small, sharp knife, split each pitta into 2 rounds. Stack the 4 rounds and make 3 crosswise cuts to form 24 pitta wedges.

On a baking sheet, arrange the pitta wedges rough sides up. With a pastry brush, lightly coat each wedge with the oil. Sprinkle the wedges evenly with the thyme, cayenne, and cheese. Bake 8–10 minutes until crisp and golden brown. Serve warm or at room temperature. Store tightly covered at room temperature for up to 2 days.

2 wholemeal pittas, 15 cm (6 in) in diameter

1½ teaspoons olive oil or sunflower oil

½ teaspoon dried thyme

¼ teaspoon cayenne pepper

2 tablespoons grated Romano or Parmesan cheese

NUTRIENT ANALYSIS FOR ONE SERVING

Calories 88	**Carbohydrates** 13 g	**Total Fat** 3 g
Protein 3 g	**Fibre** 2 g	**Saturated Fat** 1 g
Sodium 157 mg	**Sugars** 0 g	**Monounsaturated Fat** 2 g
Cholesterol 3 mg		**Polyunsaturated Fat** 0 g

INGREDIENTS & TECHNIQUES

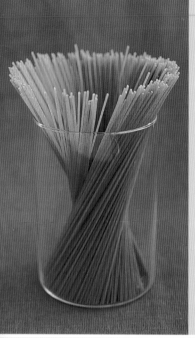

AL DENTE

Italian for "to the tooth", *al dente* refers to the firm texture traditionally desired in boiled dried pasta. It should not be hard at the centre, but it should offer slight resistance when bitten. The best way to determine when it has reached this stage is by tasting the pasta near the end of its cooking time. Depending on its shape, most dried pasta requires 8 to 12 minutes of boiling.

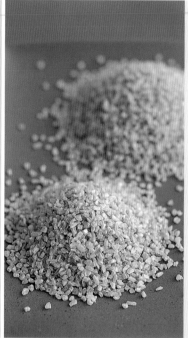

BULGUR WHEAT

A staple in the Middle East, bulgur comes from whole-wheat kernels that have been partially steamed, dried, and then cracked. It's widely available in a range of granulations, from a coarse grain for pilaf to a fine grinding for tabbouleh. Commonly used in salads, soups, and fillings, bulgur requires only brief soaking in water or a few minutes of cooking to bring out its nutty flavour.

BRAISING

This technique involves searing over high heat, then simmering in a tightly covered pot. Browning and long cooking develop deep flavours, while low heat and moisture coax tougher cuts of meat into tenderness. Braising helps swell the starches in firm vegetables like carrots, winter squash, and sweet potatoes, and soften the tough fibres in dark greens such as kale and spring greens.

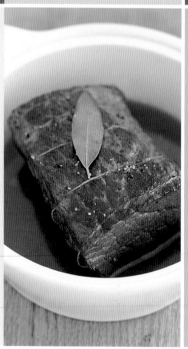

CAPERS

The flower buds of a spiny Mediterranean shrub, capers have a pleasantly pungent flavour. They lend a bright piquancy to a wide variety of sauces, salads, and dips. Although they're commonly available pickled in vinegar, capers that have been packed in salt retain the best flavour and texture. Briefly soak pickled capers or rinse salted ones in cold water to remove excess salt before using.

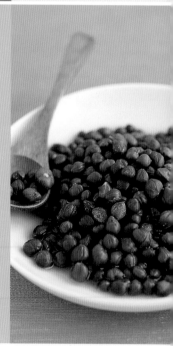

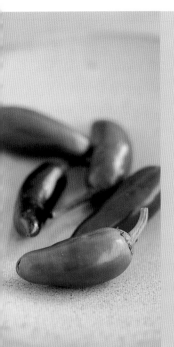

CHILLIES

A staple around the world, chillies – hot peppers – vary widely in shape, colour, flavour, and heat levels. Most ripen from green to bright red, sweetening as they redden. Generally speaking, the smaller the chilli the hotter it is, but beware as there are a few exceptions to the rule. Roast them first to bring out their smoky, earthy flavour and then add them to soups, stews, and sauces.

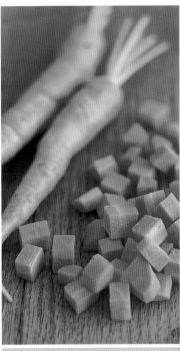

CHOPPING & DICING VEGETABLES

Cutting vegetables into even pieces when chopping ensures even cooking. Dicing is more precise since the vegetables are cut into neat cubes. This cut is often used in recipes, when appearance is important. To dice, first cut vegetables into thick slices with a large knife. Stack the slices, cut long pieces, then cut the pieces crosswise into cubes.

COOKING DRIED BEANS

For a fine texture, soak dried beans in water for at least 8 hours or overnight; drain and rinse. In a large pot, combine beans and water to cover by 5 cm (2 in). Bring the beans to a boil, cover partially, and simmer over low heat 40 to 50 minutes until tender. Continue as directed in the recipe. Most varieties yield about 275–350 g (10–20 oz) cooked beans for every 100 g (4 oz) dried.

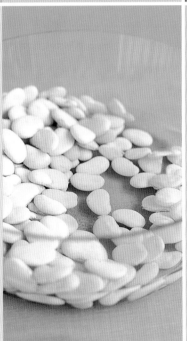

LINSEED

These tiny seeds, varying in colour from pale gold to brown, have a nutty flavour that blends well in baked goods or cereals. For the best flavour and nutrient value, grind whole linseed in a coffee grinder, food processor, or blender. Whole linseed can be stored indefinitely at room temperature, but once ground, it should be kept in an airtight container in the refrigerator.

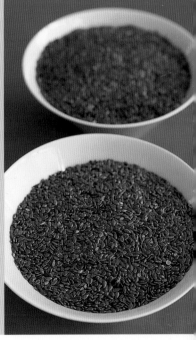

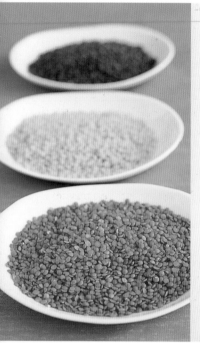

LENTILS

A staple in the Middle East for 8,000 years, lentils are now available in dozens of kinds grown around the world. Varieties include the common brown lentil found in most supermarkets, dark green Le Puy lentils from France, yellow lentils from India, and the small red lentils of Egypt. Although always dried, they do not require presoaking and cook to tenderness in only 20 to 30 minutes.

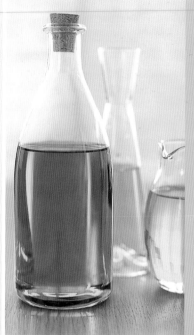

OLIVE OIL

Essential to Mediterranean cuisine, olive oils can be bright green and peppery or mellow gold and slightly sweet. Extra-virgin olive oil, the highest quality grade, retains the most colour and flavour, but reserve it for sauces and quick sautés, as it loses character at even moderate temperatures. Regular olive oil, lighter in flavour and colour, holds up well to high-heat cooking, such as grilling.

NUTMEG, WHOLE

Native to Indonesia, nutmeg has a warm, sweet-spicy flavour that marries well with spinach, fish, meat fillings, milk-based dishes, and many desserts. Because its aromatic oils dissipate quickly once the seed is ground, try to use whole nutmeg whenever possible. Although special nutmeg graters ensure the finest shavings, a fine-holed or Microplane grater also works well.

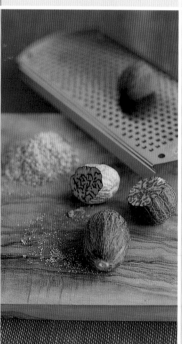

PEELING MANGOES

To peel and dice a mango, stand it on one of its narrow ends. Cut the mango off-centre, just grazing one side of the stone. Repeat on the other side. Score the cut side of the two lobes in a grid without piercing the peel. Press the mango lobes inside out and slice off the cubes of fruit near the peel. Remove the peel from the fruit around the stone, then cut the fruit away from the stone.

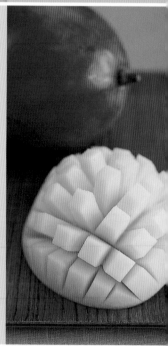

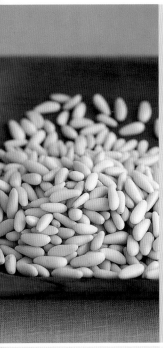

PINE NUTS

Also known as pine kernels, these pale, slender nuts are laboriously harvested from the cones of pine trees indigenous to southern Europe and the southern United States. Ground or whole, raw or toasted, they lend richness to a wide variety of savoury and sweet dishes, from classic Italian pesto and Mexican sweets to simple salads and pastas. They're especially good toasted.

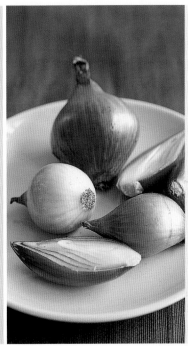

SHALLOTS

Diminutive members of the onion family, shallots grow in small clusters much like garlic. Their papery, reddish brown skin covers white flesh tinged with pink or purple. Although layered like onions, with a similar pungent aroma, they are valued for their more delicate flavour, which is particularly good in sauces and vinaigrettes. Store shallots in a cool, dark place with good air circulation.

SESAME OIL

Made from toasted sesame seeds, dark sesame oil has a rich amber colour and an intense, nutty flavour. Clear, refined sesame oils are better for high-heat cooking, but dark oils offer more flavour, even in tiny amounts. Look for them in Asian markets or the international section of supermarkets. More perishable than other oils, dark sesame oil is best stored in the refrigerator.

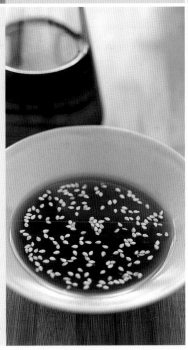

FRESH SOYA BEANS

Also known as edamame, soya beans picked still in their pods retain a bright green colour and a fresh, nutty flavour. Left whole, they can be boiled or steamed for a snack. Shelled, they're enjoyed like garden peas in vegetable dishes, soups, or purées. Look for soya beans during summer in farmers' markets or year-round in the freezers of health-food stores and Asian markets.

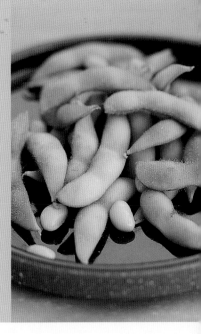

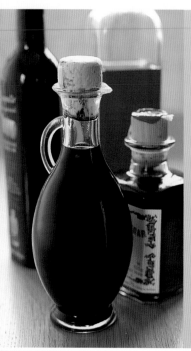

SPECIALTY VINEGARS

French for "sour wine", vinegar forms when bacteria turn a fermented liquid into a weak solution of acetic acid. Red wine, white wine, balsamic, and sherry vinegars are among the best for cooking, as they display traits of the wines from which they are made, along with a sourness that makes them valuable in balancing flavours. Look for unfiltered, top-quality aged vinegars.

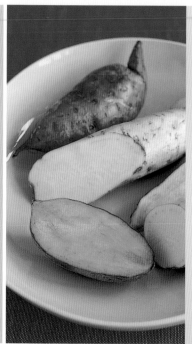

SWEET POTATOES

Although often confused with yams, sweet potatoes have a sweeter flavour and less starchy flesh. They are excellent baked whole, roasted or braised with a honey or maple syrup glaze, or mashed with a touch of cinnamon or nutmeg. Shop for sweet potatoes free of dark blemishes. Store in a cool, dark, well-ventilated place but avoid refrigerating them, as cold temperatures will alter their flavour.

SWEET ONIONS

The best-known varieties of these onions include brown (or cooking onions) and Spanish onions. Spanish onions are larger and have a milder flavour. When they are finished in May, the same types of onion are imported from the Southern hemisphere. Onions with white papery skins are sometimes available and are even sweeter, as are red onions.

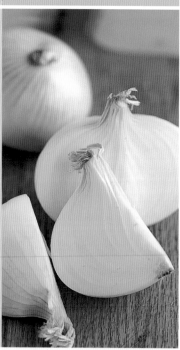

TOASTING NUTS

Cooking nuts until they are golden deepens their flavour and improves their texture. You can toast nuts on a baking sheet in a 170°C (325°F) oven or by stirring them in a small, dry, non-stick frying pan over medium-high heat. Cook them about 10 minutes until they're fragrant and golden in colour. Don't overcook them, as they will become bitter when scorched.

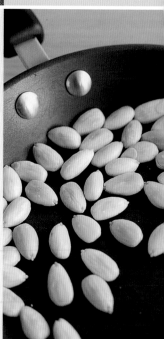

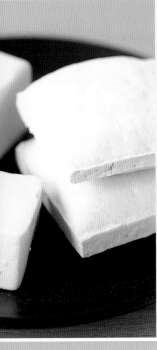

TOFU

Soya milk, made from cooked soya beans, forms tofu when curdled and pressed into blocks. Although bland, plain tofu readily absorbs flavours from marinades and sauces. The smooth texture of silken tofu is ideal for soups and for puréeing. Firm tofu, denser and coarser in texture, holds together well for stir-frying and grilling. To store tofu, submerge it in cold water and refrigerate.

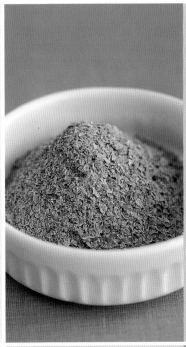

WHEAT BRAN AND WHEAT GERM

During the milling of wheat, the kernel's outer covering, known as the bran, and its tiny embryo, the germ, are usually both removed. Sold in health-food stores and most supermarkets, wheat bran and wheat germ add nutrient value to cereals, casseroles, fillings, and baked goods. Unless the germ is defatted, it should be stored in an airtight container in the refrigerator.

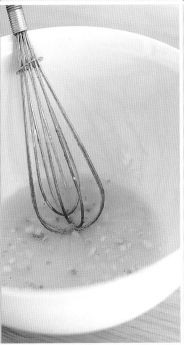

VINAIGRETTE

Making a vinaigrette involves little more than whisking together a small amount of oil, vinegar, salt, pepper, and perhaps an aromatic ingredient, such as garlic, shallots, a dab of prepared mustard, or some chopped fresh herbs. In addition to dressing salads, a vinaigrette can be used as a marinade before roasting, a basting liquid at the barbecue, or a sauce for steamed vegetables.

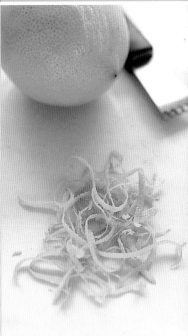

ZEST

The thin outer peel of citrus fruits, known as the zest, is rich in aromatic oils. A fine-holed or Microplane grater will shred the zest into delicate shavings for marinades or rubs. Use a zester to create thin, elegant strips for garnish. Take care not to cut or grate into the white, pulpy pith that lies just beneath the outer peel, as it has a spongy texture and an unpleasantly bitter flavour.

INDEX

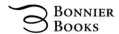

BONNIER BOOKS

Appledram Barns
Birdham Road
Chichester, West Sussex
PO20 7EQ

AMERICAN MEDICAL ASSOCIATION

Executive Vice President,
  Chief Executive Officer: Michael D. Maves, M.D.
Senior Vice President,
  Publishing and Business Services: Robert A. Musacchio, Ph.D.
Vice President, Business Products: Anthony J. Frankos
Chief Operations Officer, AMA Press: Mary Lou White
Managing Editor: Donna Kotulak
Writer: Pam Brick
Editors: Robin Husayko, Steve Michaels
Copy Editor: Reuben Rios
Art Editor: Mary Ann Albanese
Medical Editor: Bonnie Chi-Lum, M.D., M.P.H.
Contributing Editor: Maryellen Westerberg, Dr.P.H., R.D., C.D.E.
Consultants: Clair M. Callan, M.D., Thomas Houston, M.D.

The recommendations and information in this book are appropriate
in most cases and current as of the date of publication. For specific
information, concerning your or a family member's medical
condition, the AMA suggests that you consult a physician.

WELDON OWEN INC.

Chief Executive Officer: John Owen
President and Chief Operating Officer: Terry Newell
Vice President International Sales: Stuart Laurence
Vice President and Creative Director: Gaye Allen
Associate Creative Director: Leslie Harrington
Associate Publisher: Val Cipollone
Managing Editor: Sheridan Warrick
Designer: Leon Yu
Cover Designer: Kelly Booth
Editorial Assistants: Mitch Goldman, Juli Vendzules
Copy Editor and Proofreader: Carrie Bradley and Desne Ahlers
Indexer: Ken DellaPenta
Production Director: Chris Hemesath
Colour Specialist: Teri Bell
Production Coordinator: Todd Rechner

The American Medical Association Diabetes Cookbook
Conceived and produced by Weldon Owen Inc.
814 Montgomery Street, San Francisco, CA 94133
Telephone: 415-291-0100 Fax: 415-291-8841

U.S. Edition originally published in 2004

First printed in 2007
10 9 8 7 6 5 4 3 2 1

ISBN: 978-1-905825-13-4
Printed by Midas Printing Limited, China

Acknowledgements
Thanks to Kyrie Forbes, Karin Skaggs, Joan Olson, and Robin Terra
for design assistance; Joseph De Leo for art direction; Suzette
Kaminsky, Kim Konecny, Erin Quon, and Dan Becker for food styling;
Joe Maer and Leigh Noë for prop styling; Kevin Kerr and Selena
Aument for assisting in the studio; and Heather Dunn, Gina Bessire,
Tanya Henry, and Jackie Mancuso for modeling.

Photographs by Sheri Giblin: pages 9 (bottom right), 13 (three at left),
14 (middle at right), 15, 16 (three at right), 25 (third from top), 26, 32,
44, 52, 55, 65, 79, 82, 85, 86, 89, 94, 110, 114, 116, 119.